Edited by

CHRISTINE DEAN
International Mental Health Network

CW01558635

A Slow Train Coming

Bringing the Mental Health Revolution to Scotland

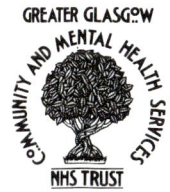

Published by: The Greater Glasgow Community and Mental Health Services NHS
                  Trust
                  Trust Headquarters
                  Gartnavel Royal Hospital
                  1055 Great Western Road
                  Glasgow G12 0XH

British Library Cataloguing in Publication Data. A catalogue record for this book is available from the British Library.

ISBN 0-9524569-0-7

The publishers are not responsible for any error of omission or fact.

Printed in Great Britain by Mackay and Inglis Limited, Glasgow, Scotland.

FOREWORD

SCOTTISH CONFERENCE ON MENTAL HEALTH

I welcome publication and wider availability of the contributions to the 1993 Scottish Conference on Mental Health. I only regret that on the day I was unable to participate and to hear at first hand the speeches and exchanges from the impressive list of participants.

I hope others, like me, will find these speeches to be both interesting and stimulating and a useful account of where we are with mental health services and where we aim to be.

The Rt Hon the Lord Fraser of Carmyllie QC
Minister for Home Affairs and Health
The Scottish Office

CONTENTS

LIST OF CONTRIBUTORS

John Basson, Principal Medical Officer, The Scottish Office, St. Andrew's House, Edinburgh EH1 3DG

Jerry Bereika, Operations Director, Lifeways Community Care, 4 Thameside Centre, Kew Bridge Road, Brentford, Middlesex TW8 0HB.

Joe Bouch, Consultant Psychiatrist, Goldenhill Resource Centre, 2 Stuart Drive, Clydebank

Tom Burns, Professor in Psychiatry, St. George's Hospitsl Medical School, Jenner Wing, Cranmer Terrace, London SW17 0RE.

Mr. Peter Campbell, Survivors Speak Out, 34 Osnaburgh Street, London NW1 3ND.

Derek Chiswick, Consultant Forensic Psychiatrist, Royal Edinburgh Hospital, Morningside Terrace, Edinburgh EH10 5HF.

Dr. Edna Conlan, MBE, Chair of United Kingdom Advocacy Network (UKAN), Premier House, 14 Cross Burgess Street, Sheffield S1 2HJ.

Laurie Davidson, Consultant in Training and Team Development in Mental Health, Brambly Wood, Hayton, Newton Abbot, South Devon TQ13 9XH.

Tim Davison, Chief Executive, Greater Glasgow Community & Mental Health Services NHS Trust, Gartnavel Royal Hospital, 1055 Great Western Road, Glasgow G12 0XH.

Christine Dean, Senior Consultant in Community Mental Health Services Development, International Mental Health Network, St. Martins House, Bull King, Birmingham B5 5DT.

Dr. Linda de Caesteker, Consultant in Public Health Medicine, Greater Glasgow Health Board, 112 Ingram Street, Glasgow G1 1ET.

Ronald J. Diamond, Medical Director, Mental Health Center of Dane County, 600 Hihland Avenue, Madison, Wisconsin, W1 53792, U.S.A.

Mr. Peter Gilroy, Director of Operations, Kent County Council, Social Services, Springfield, Maidstone, Kent ME14 2LW (also Mental Health Task Force).

J. Greenwood, Consultant Psychiatrist, Community Drug Problem Service, Royal Edinburgh Hospital, Morningside Terrance, Edinburgh EH10 5HF.

Mary C. Hartnoll, Director of Social Work, Strathclyde Regional Council, Strathclyde House, 20 India Street, Glasgow G2 4PF.

Gregor Henderson, Community Services Development Manager, Homewood NHS Trust, Homewood House, Guildford Road, Chertsey, Surrey KT16 0QA.

John H. Henderson, Consultant in Mental Health, Herveys Cottage, 56 Church Way, Weston Favell, Northampton NN3 3BX, President, European Regional Council of the World Federation for Mental Health, 110 Franklin Street, Brussels B-1040, Belgium.

Nigel Henderson, Research & Development Manager, Penumbra, Gogar Park, 167 Glasgow Road Edinburgh EH12 9BG.

Peter Hoare, Senior Lecturer, Department of Child and Family Psychiatry, 3 Rillbank Terrace, Edinburgh EH9 1LL.

John Hoult, Consultant Psychiatrist, Northern Birmingham Mental Health Trust, Newbridge House, Yardley Green Hospital, Yardley Green Road, Birmingham B9 5PX.

Anne Jarvie, Chief Nursing Officer, The Scottish Office, St. Andrew's House, Edinburgh EH1 3DE.

John B. Jenkins, Senior Consultant in Community Mental Health Services Development, International Mental Health Network, St. Martins House, Bull Ring, Birmingham B5 5DT.

Christine Kirk, Consultant Psychogeriatrician, Bootham Park Hospital, York YO3 7BY.

John Loudon, Clinical Director, Edinburgh District, Royal Edinburgh Hospital, Morningside Terrace, Edinburgh EH10 5HF.

Donald Lyons, Consultant Psychogeriatrician, Leverndale Hospital, 510 Crookston Road, Glasgow G53 7TU.

Bill Moyes, Director of Purchasing Strategy, Management Executive, The Scottish Office, St. Andrew's House, Edinburgh EH1 3DG.

Peter Millar, Director, Richmond Fellowship, 9 Sandyford Place, Glasgow G3 7NB.

Isobel Morris, Head of Department of Clinical Psychology, Guy's and St. Thomas' Hospital Trust, Mental Health Unit, York Clinic, 117 Borough High Street, London SE1 1NP.

Lawrence Nugent, Glasgow Association for Mental Health (GAMH) , Melrose House, 15/23 Cadogan Street, Glasgow G2 6PQ.

Mr. Jim Read, Survivors Speak Out, 34 Osnaburgh Street, London NW1 3ND.

B. Ritson, Consultant Psychiatrist, Alcohol Problems Clinic, Royal Edinburgh Hospital, Morningside Terrace, Edinburgh EH10 5HF.

Mr. Martin Sime, Director, Scottish Council for Voluntary Organisations, 18/19 Claremont Crescent, Edinburgh EH7 4QD.

Brian Smith, Scottish Users Network (SUN), c/o Edinburgh Association for Mental Health, 40 Shandwick Place, Edinburgh EH2 4RT.

Professor Chris Thompson, Professor in Psychiatry & Registrar, Royal College of Psychiatrists, 17 Belgrave Square, London SW1X 8PG.

D. Tonak, MBE, Advisor on Services for Mentally Disordered Offenders, Winston Churchill Memorial Trust, 15 Queen's Gate Terrace, London SW7 5PR.

Andrew Webster, Purchasing Commissioner of Priority Services, Greater Glasgow Health Board, 112 Ingram Street, Glasgow G1 1ET.

Richard Williams, Director, NHS Health Advisory Service, Sutherland House, 29-37 Brighton Road, Sutton, Surrey SM2 5AN.

KEYNOTE ADDRESS FROM THE SCOTTISH OFFICE

BILL MOYES

What I want to do is to set out the Government's vision for good quality mental health services and to say something about how we hope to achieve it. The Government's aim is that mental health service should, by the end of the decade, have 4 main characteristics. **First** that they should be patient centred. **Second** that they should be of high quality. **Third** that they be effective and **finally** that they should be efficient in the use of resources.

What has to be done to achieve these objectives? First of all services have to be developed which are genuinely community based and which are not institutionally based. In Scotland there is still quite a bias towards institutionally based services. To shift the balance resources need to move away from institutional provision and towards community based provision.

The second thing that needs to be achieved is a service which sees people as individuals, and which attempts to meet their needs rather than letting them make do with what can be selected from a pretty restricted range of services. So we need to know how to tailor the services we offer to meet the needs of the individual.

The third thing that needs to be done is to develop further joint planning and working by different agencies involved in the provision of mental health services; joint planning to ensure that services compliment each other, and that resources are used to best effect and joint working to ensure that the client is unaware of the boundaries between different service providers. If the service is really going to be patient centred and of high quality it should not be the client that negotiates the package of care.

This is not to say that every agency has to try and do everything; different agencies have different roles, different responsibilities, they work within different legal frameworks which have to be respected. Ways of joint working have to be devised so that the package of services that the client gets appears to the client to be completely seamless, and delivered without the client being aware of the negotiations and machinations that inevitably go on when different agencies are trying to work together.

The fourth thing which has to be achieved is services which are neither excessive nor inadequate. "Excessive" may be a slightly strange word to use but I think it needs to be recognised that there are some people, certainly at present and I guess in the future, who may be provided with a level of care which exceeds the needs they have and that they are therefore being made dependant by that inappropriate pattern of service.

The consequence of that is that other people will be getting inadequate services because of this misapplication of resources. It is important to make sure that the services the clients get are properly balanced with their needs.

Finally, it is necessary to achieve a pattern of service that aims to prevent admission to long-stay facilities and aims to return people to the community with proper support services. Proper programmes of rehabilitation built in from the outset of the provision of services are necessary.

Close co-operation between the primary and secondary care sectors is necessary, with the secondary care sector reaching into the community to support the primary care services. Primary care includes not only primary health care, but social work services and many of the services that housing agencies can offer.What pattern of service would be generated if this vision came to pass?

What pattern of service should be engineered to achieve this vision?

Two or 3 years ago under the previous Chief Executive of the NHS, the purpose and values of the NHS began to be thought about, in the process that eventually led to the publication of the Patient's Charter and the Framework For Action.

It was concluded that the first responsibility for the NHS was to improve health and secondly, to deliver high quality health care. This has to be as true in the area of mental health as for acute services and I do not think we can regard the improvement of health as uniquely an issue for acute service providers and purchasers.

So, we need to try to get in place programmes of preventative work where it is relevant for mental health conditions such as depression, and these programmes need to involve agencies other than health agencies. There are a wide range of agencies that can play a part in offering these kind of services, and we need to try and identify where they are relevant and see if we can make them happen.

We also need to develop primary care services which diagnose and treat effectively a wider range of mental health problems than they perhaps tackle at present. To do that they need to be properly supported by outreach services from the secondary care sector, and again they need to involve other agencies. Primary health care should not be seen as working in a vacuum. For example, how much depression and neurosis might be capable of being treated entirely in the primary care sector if there were social workers or counsellors working with general practitioners (GPs) or community psychiatric nurses working in Health Centres? More emphasis should be given to developing these kind of services, to investigating how effective they might be, and whether a different pattern of service could produce a better and different outcome for patients.

More community mental health and mental handicap teams involving both health care and social work professionals need to be developed. Some of these teams may be consultant led but perhaps not all; that will depend on the kind of needs that these teams are trying to meet. The development of a wide range of day facilities is required and more of them should be jointly purchased rather than clients being segregated into NHS clients and social work clients with different services being provided in different locations.

Some of the boundaries should be slightly blurred so that the same facility jointly purchased, jointly operated can serve a wider range of clients. The department would like to see the development of adequate assessment facilities with truly multi-disciplinary assessment teams working to agreed protocols and timetables.

Adequate in-patient facilities should be available for those who really need them, for patients for example who from time to time suffer acute breakdowns and need short in-patient stays. The Government would like to see more of the facilities they need and would like to see them located on the site of district general hospitals and not in separate segregated facilities. Long-stay accommodation will be required for people whose behaviour simply cannot be managed in the community or whose clinical needs require long-term in-patient provision supervised by a consultant. Again for these patients the objective is that facilities will not be segregated from communities but located within communities.

Adequate services should be developed for particular groups of people, those who abuse alcohol and drugs, people who need the services of forensic psychiatry, children and adolescents and so on. The Government would like to see a wide range of domiciliary services jointly purchased and provided by health, housing and social work and a wide range of residential facilities offering different kinds of service to different kinds of patients, and involving health, social work and housing providers and the public and private sectors working in co-operation.

It is also important to develop support for carers who after all are probably the biggest single service provider. Some health boards in Scotland and a number of district health authorities in England are now offering training programmes to carers to help them to care effectively. Support groups are developing in a number of areas and 24 hour, 7 day a week respite care facilities not necessarily admitting patients for 2 or 3 weeks but sometimes simply admitting overnight so that the carer can get a break, or providing someone to turn to if there are difficulties in the night. Increasingly carers are being involved by purchasers and providers in planning services and that is something to be encouraged.

If that is the vision seen by the Government of what a quality patient-centred cost-effective mental health service should be like, how does the existing situation compare? The answer is patchy. Starting at the level of planning, my assessment is that the overall situation is getting much better. Two years ago there might have been criticism about how community care and mental health planning was developing, but not today. A lot of good work is going on. In some cases the plans still represent separate but well co-ordinated streams of activity and that is fine - a big improvement on the past. Here and there are the beginnings of truly meshed together plans that represent exciting developments with joint planning and joint working.

Seen from St Andrew's House, community care and mental health planning still places too much emphasis on inputs, rather than concentrating on the kind of targets that the service will have to try and achieve and the kind of outcomes that must be achieved for clients. There is a general recognition that planning needs to move towards what is going to be achieved rather than what is going to go into the system. Most important of all under the heading of planning there is now - at least as seen from my desk - a much higher level of shared concept between health, social work and housing, than would have been the case a few years ago. There are many more fully shared agendas. Housing in particular I think is much more involved in the process of developing mental health and community care services than was the case 3 or 4 years ago.

At the level of purchasing more needs to be done. Health boards still need to develop a greater capacity for planning and purchasing mental health services. Some boards have quite strong purchasing teams, but even where purchasers do have expertise in the area of mental health they are still not giving enough attention to the specialised components of a mental health service, for example forensic psychiatry or child and adolescent psychiatry services.

There is also too little effort going into defining outcome measures for mental health services. I recognise this is difficult, but in acute services a lot of activity has gone on in the last 18 months or so under the auspices of CRAG (Clinical Resource and Audit Group) and against expectation, good progress has been made.

Outcome measures need to be developed as part of dictating the agenda for developing information systems. We need to know what the outcome is now for the patients treated by the service and how it could be improved in the future, and we need to know what information to collect to measure such outcomes.

Better and joint information systems need to be developed compared to those current in the acute sector. The information available in mental health services and in community care is limited, and what it tells you is often ineffective and incomplete.

Service delivery is more difficult for someone from the Scottish Office to offer any good judgement on, but from that perspective services do not yet always appear to be tailored to the needs of the individual and resources are not always used as effectively as they might. Sometimes there are overlaps between services and sometimes there are gaps. The cost of delivering a particular service can vary widely across the country.

The policy of care in the community in its latest manifestation has not been in place for very long but already there are signs of the development of a real and lasting will on the part of different agencies to work together not just at the level of planning but at the level of delivering services. There is the emergence of a very good and useful joint understanding of what different agencies are trying to achieve, the constraints under which they operate and how by working together they can achieve more than by working separately.

Where do we go from here? Firstly, there is a desperate need to move away from our existing long-stay institutions and get Health Boards, Local Authorities and housing agencies planning together to achieve that. They need to identify and close those institutions that in the longer term do not have a role in the provision of the mental health services of the future. They need to work together to build up the community based facilities that will allow the institutional provision to be closed. Health, social work and housing need jointly to channel resources to achieve the transition from institutional care to community care in a reasonable timescale; there is a lot of evidence to suggest that if an institution is going to close and if the pattern of service is going to move to a community based one, the transition should be achieved over 3 or 4 years rather than 8 or 10 years.

The Government is looking to see the transfer of something like 600 patients or places from institutions into the community in Scotland each year. The amount of in-patient facilities that the NHS provides for the frail elderly will also contract although the scale of that contraction has yet to be properly assessed. If that kind of transition were to be achieved we would see a reduction of perhaps 30% or so by the end of the decade or by early next century in the volume of institutional provision. The early evidence that we have is that actually a rather faster rate of contraction seems likely as health boards, housing agencies and local authorities really do work together.

The second main issue is the need to build and provide a range of facilities in the community. Singularly important is effective assessment services to ascertain the needs of all mentally ill people within a locally defined area. Local authorities have been given guidance on procedures and the resources necessary to carry out the assessments. It is local authorities who are in the lead in seeking and co-ordinating views and in arranging the provision of services. For someone who is thought to have a mental health problem, local authorities should be seeking advice from medical and other professionals. Local authorities are now getting to grips with these very new procedures and responsibilities but it is too soon to be clear about what real progress is being made and whether any different arrangements or support from Government is needed. Sufficient places need to be secured in local authority homes, sheltered housing, supported lodgings or similar forms of provision for adults with a mental illness who need residential care that is not hospital care.

Well trained and co-ordinated mental health teams from health and social work backgrounds are needed to support mentally ill people in their own homes, with the capacity to respond to crisis and to provide emergency out of hours services. The same multi-disciplinary mental illness services are required for the elderly with dementia in the community and these need to be backed up by appropriate specialist in-patient NHS facilities for elderly people who need that kind of care. There needs to be appropriate specialist provision for groups with particular psychological problems like children and adolescents.

Training is another important issue when we are considering a contraction in the long-stay NHS sector. Staff need to be retrained to provide alternative forms of care and to help them to move from present employment to alternatives. Facilities to provide training and education to the care staff who work in institutions and who are working in the community need to be available and extended to carers and relatives.

How is this transition going to be achieved and what kind of levers do we have now and how effective are they being? The first is bridging finance. Since this was introduced in 1991 we have made available a total of something like £63M in bridging finance. Just about half of that has already been taken up and has secured the transfer of hundreds of patients into the community and prevented the unnecessary admission or re-admission to hospital of many more.

At the moment there is still £8M worth of bridging finance available in the current financial year (1993-1994). There is £13M available next year and £15M the year after that. Ministers' current intention is to maintain bridging finance at around the level of £15M per annum, so long as it continues to achieve the objectives the Government has set.

Bridging finance was generally welcomed, when it was introduced and it is a very important part of securing the transition from institutional to community care. It is disappointing therefore that the bids against the resources that we have available are currently running at relatively low levels. Health boards and local authorities should be encouraged to work up detailed proposals and submit them to the Scottish Office.

The other lever the Scottish Office has is the transfer of the resources from health boards to local authorities. Bridging finance is meant to facilitate the process of transferring people into the community and resource transfers are intended to help secure their placement.

As patients transfer, the lead responsibility for their care transfers from the health board to local authority. The government has made it quite clear that where this happens the transfer will be accompanied by a transfer of cash from the health board to the local authority. The objective is not only to stimulate the development of places in the community but also to provide community based services for patients who would otherwise have to be inappropriately admitted to long-stay NHS care. This important process of transferring people into the community will only work if health boards make realistic and adequate transfer of resources to local authorities to meet the new responsibilities. The previous Chief Executive, Don Cruickshank, talked about a transfer of the order of £150M to £200M over the next decade and that is still the view of the Scottish Office. I also think it is essential for health boards to be open with local authorities about this process, about what resources will be released by closing institutions or by transferring responsibility for particular groups of patients. We are not looking for closed book negotiations, we are looking for openness and honesty and joint discussions between health and social work about how the resources released can be used most effectively.

Another lever is the development of joint purchasing. There will be patients whose needs will never be capable of being neatly compartmentalised into health care or social care. At times their needs will be for social care and at other times health care needs will predominate. To provide effectively for patients like this the Government wants to see health boards and local authorities pooling the resources that each currently devotes to the long-term care of the elderly, the elderly with dementia and people with mental illness and learning disability. Having pooled their resources the agencies concerned can then decide jointly on how the available resource might best be used to meet the needs of clients and patients. One of the big things that our new Chief Executive , Geoff Scaife, said to me shortly after he arrived was that he thought he had operated this system very effectively when he was Regional General Manager in Merseyside. As I understand it he and the local Director of Social Services met together to discuss the resources which they were both currently devoting to mental health and community care services and decided annually how both allocations of resources were going to be used. They did not always purchase jointly, quite often they contracted in parallel because of legal difficulties with jointly agreed specifications and very tightly specified services, but the main thing was that they worked closely together in defining the resources available and in deciding how they should be allocated. This is certainly a more effective way of securing services than separate activity.

Finally let me just mention the mental illness specific grant introduced in April 1991 to try to bolster the few facilities in the community that were currently provided for people with mental illnesses. There are now something like 250 projects which are receiving a grant from a total budget of £10M. These projects are directed mainly towards preventing the need for people in the community to enter hospital. This year the Scottish Office urged authorities to develop projects which linked with health boards' projects to assist people moving from long-stay institutions to the community. Some projects which have come into the Scottish Office fit that criterion and we expect that increasingly to be the case as local authorities are encouraged to develop such projects with health boards and housing authorities. The figures at the Scottish Office suggest that mental illness specific grant assisted around 25,000 people in the community last year, and it is hoped that this number will continue to rise as the level of grant continues to increase.

THE CHANGING ROLE OF PURCHASERS

JOHN BASSON

I think it is important to start from the position that the purchaser/provider split is not well developed in Scotland with regard to mental health. We have to establish the separation of purchasing from providing. A Health Board cannot concentrate on realising the potential of purchasing if it is also responsible for running the local hospitals. We must make progress towards establishing NHS trusts and in negotiations with Local Authorities and voluntary agencies. The roles of each need to be clearly defined.

In this context I would like to use as a framework a speech given by Dr Brian Mawhinney, Minister for Health in the earlier part of this year. He made 5 points.

Firstly purchasing must reach out to the future, not simply replicate the past; it will involve a shift away from the status quo. This is self-evident in so far as we are moving not only to a purchaser/provider split but away from large institutions and into community care. We are establishing a partnership both within and outside the health service. We must appreciate this is a process which is underway, it is inevitable, it is appropriate, and it will require a lot of goodwill.

Secondly an element of competition between providers, and also between purchasers is vital for change. This can be seen in 2 ways:-

1. The competition to provide innovative, quality, value for money services. One area services compares itself to another. They are not close enough to compete for clients/patients but they are similar enough to compare the methods used, costs and other factors. This presumes the availability of information.

2. Competition for clients/patients. This will be more obvious with LA and the voluntary/private provision. All should be encouraged to put forward plans for addressing the needs of the population and improving the quality of provision.

Thirdly there must be shared purchasing between health boards and all GPs (including Fundholders); all family doctors must be closely involved in the purchasing process.

Fourthly contracting between purchasers and providers is a powerful mechanism for change, but it needs development. Doctors and nurses must become more closely involved in the contracting process. It is important to stress that with the mental health services a wide range of professionals should be consulted depending on the client group. Those colleagues who have population information - epidemiologically based as well as financial must also be consulted.

Fifthly purchasing is about developing and managing relationships. Its successful development will require effective leadership and commitment. This is a key area. For the process of community care to be successful health/social work/housing and voluntary plus private agencies must talk, co-operate. plan and manage together. Those who cannot work in this way are obviously unsuitable members of a purchasing team.

These points should be examined.

Some fundamental issues with respect to purchasing came from a ministerial speech earlier in the year.

What is purchasing? For over 40 years the NHS in Scotland has been provider-driven and no more so than in mental health. We now wish to move it to be a purchaser-driven organisation. Given the radical nature of this move 2 points in the process have to be remembered. Firstly the provider bases must be protected. Secondly the purchaser must be helped to develop skills to be good at the job.

In the future fully fledged purchasing will have the following attributes.

* *It is not about directly managing services.* I have already mentioned the development of Trusts - this is important. I perceive that both purchasers and providers in the health services want to do each others jobs at the present time. This is sometimes from a sense of frustration but also from a failure to adopt a new thinking approach. Providers write sometimes the strategy the purchaser should have written probably because of a lack of expertise in the purchasing staff and providers deciding where and in what buildings future services will be provided - again because both sides do not understand the split in tasks. Occasionally there is a feeling of threat which causes people to do a job which is not theirs.

* *It is not about protecting the income of local providers at all costs.* It will take some time to come to terms with resource transfer and operating a smaller budget in mental health services. The final product will, however, be more based on professional skill and expertise. I also think that social workers - LA, voluntary agency and private agency employed - will have to adjust to the responsibilities of caring for groups of mentally ill and handicapped in the community - initially the beds in hospital remain during the dual running process with bridging finance but ultimately after resource transfer there is no way back. We must plan carefully, train well and cover contingencies in plans.

* *It is not about localising services on grounds of access alone without regard to other aspects of quality and value for money.* This has been an issue with regard to forensic psychiatry services for those patients requiring special care in a secure environment. Many people would wish to move from the state hospital at Carstairs to a more locally based service for this small but significant group. After weighing up the quality, value for money and locally based arguments the Scottish office decided on the redevelopment of

one site at Carstairs for the group and the complimentary services locally to be examined with a view to improvement, to keep in step with Carstairs developments.

* *Equally it is not about imposing requirements on providers in the expectation that they will simply get on with it.* In some places the providers are the weak link in the chain and will need a lot of work before they can embark on the radical changes proposed; this is underway. There also may be specific areas where a purchaser/provider liaison to plan a strategy are important - eg drug misuse services, alcohol problem services etc. The local authority should also be involved as often as it can provide the basis for the development.

* *Purchasing I must stress is not a recipe for maintaining the status quo.* We have said this before. Sometimes the purchasing team will need to be brave. There are vested interests against change. Inefficiency and out-dated working methods can provide an easy living.

What services should be purchased? These must include: Acute and assessment services, long term care for those with severe behavioural problems or high dependency due to complex clinical difficulties, outreach services - eg resource centres, special secure facilities.

We should be clear about the services that will be provided by health. These should be agreed with the partners. The GPs should be clear about the availability of mental health services for the community based patient. LA social work services should appreciate and agree the target for health-run in-patient beds.

What should be the balance between competition and collaboration in purchasing?

This is a developing and changing field. At this time we need considerable collaboration so that both providers and purchasers can define their roles and start to perform them in the mental health field effectively.

What do purchasers have to do to be effective? Purchasers will need to cover the following 7 stepping stones for effective purchasing;-

A strategic view: This requires a vision which is shared and agreed between social work and health with housing and voluntary agencies playing a part, knowledge about how to make it happen, yardsticks of success, and systems for recording what is done and what needs to be done. All of these elements are part of the joint planning.

Robust contracts: These are early days in contracting mental health services. It will be necessary to develop the information base before robust contracting is achieved. Things will change over the years as the knowledge base improves. In this purchasers must endeavour to find staff who can collect the required information and create the systems. Providers are also involved in this process.

At present needs assessment figures for an authority are still produced by extrapolating from a textbook (usually Goldberg & Huxley) to the purchasers area rather than collecting the information on the ground. This will take time to improve and more collaboration at all levels will be required and with outside agencies. Issues of confidentiality and use of shared data have to be resolved.

The other stepping stones are:- knowledge based decisions, responsiveness to local people, mature relations with providers, local alliances and organisational fitness.

Following these 7 stepping stones there are 7 imperatives:-

Better working between purchasers and providers - Purchasers should have 3 aims they hope to achieve through providers.

*   They must buy to improve people's health by targeting resources on effective ways of delivering clinical care and promoting health.

*   They must buy to improve the quality of health care, making it more responsive to the needs and wishes of people.

*   They must buy to ensure that as many people as possible receive high quality care from what available resources can provide.

Involvement of doctors and nurses in the contracting process. I will use doctors as an example here - Dialogue with doctors is essential in developing services and achieving health gain objectives because managers are simply not competent to make some of the judgements required. Realism in contracts can be achieved only if they take into account doctors' views on clinical need and practice, workload planning and medical developments. The commitment of doctors is required to develop necessary guidelines for regulating activity if in-year pressures are encountered. Access to the clinical audit process can inform both purchasers and providers on the effectiveness of interventions on quality of service. Each professional group can undertake this process.

Realism about activity and the impact of change. It is important that purchasers are realistic about the volumes of service to be purchased. and that they consider the predictability and impact of change upon themselves, other purchasers and other providers. They must ensure that there are no surprises - an inadequate period of notice can be no excuse for the absence of ongoing dialogue. Inform doctors, nurses and other professionals clearly about the rationale for change and be committed to working towards it. It takes time and effort to achieve this level of co-operation, but it is central to the job.

Involvement of local authorities, social work and housing, voluntary and private agencies: Proposals for change should be shared with the local community and ideas for change also sought from them and new services developed jointly.

Appropriate contracts: In order to achieve this purchasers must listen to patients, know what they want to achieve (identify health targets), ensure service contracts relate to what they want to achieve, make better use of available information about effectiveness and outcome measures, use contracts to engage providers in health promotion, use local clinical audit and establish challenging efficiency targets to create space for improving health and quality.

Purchasers must also examine how patients are treated and obtain the patients views. They should ensure that all the relevant patients rights and standards are drawn firmly through contracts and should specify how they plan to develop and improve local standards. They must publish the standards and progress in achieving them for public consumption, ensure compliance with national waiting times targets, and set targets for out-patients waiting times.

Robust information on prices and activity: Purchasers need to be well informed about what services are available from which providers and at what levels of effectiveness, efficiency and quality, they need to use/want information to challenge existing providers and seek out new sources of supply. Providers need to know that their activities are contestable and that they are under pressure from better-performing providers.

Purchasers need a cool-headed assessment of how the new system is working in practice - sadly, often difficult to obtain. There needs to be greater clarity about roles, responsibilities and relationships above the level of purchasers and providers. That is relationships with the Scottish office, local authority and social work committee. A change in management plan which moves forward without diverting attention from good management practice.

Effective Monitoring: This needs to be shared. It needs to be timely. Purchasers need to be sensitive to a provider's capacity to generate data and they need to have the capacity to use the data. Action expected of everyone has to be understood and agreed by all and the monitoring process has to be transparent with no ambiguity.

REFERENCE

Purchasing for Health. A Framework for Action.

Speeches by Dr B Mawhinney and Sir Duncan Nichol. NHS Management Executive April/May 1993 available from: The Health Publications Unit, Heywood Stores Distribution Centre, Manchester Road, Heywood, Lancashire OL10 2PX.

INTERNATIONAL PERSPECTIVES OF COMMUNITY MENTAL HEALTH SERVICES

JOHN B. JENKINS

INTRODUCTION

Firstly to place community mental health services in the context of history. Until the late eighteenth century, in England most people with mental health problems were supported in the community. They were not the object of any particular benefit or specialized care, but were treated in the same way as other dependent people, the "needy and worthy poor", which included the senile, the incurably ill, and people with physical disabilities.

For the most part relatives received temporary or permanent financial assistance from the parish, though some private charities provided almshouses, which were at first no more than substitute households. Efforts were made to keep mentally ill people in the local community by providing their relatives or others who were prepared to care for them with permanent pensions for their support. Only in a very small minority of places were "dangerous and troublesome lunatics" segregated from society in specialised "houses of correction".

The advancing industrialisation and commercialisation of the economy, in the nineteenth century, produced profound changes to society. Small landholders were squeezed out by the enclosures, servants became labourers, and anyone who could not work became a greater burden both on the family and on the parish.

This prompted an increasingly institutional response to the relief of poverty - notably with the increasing numbers of workhouses being built. Living conditions within them were intended to be so unattractive that only the genuinely needy would submit to this form of relief.

The growing market in labour made it necessary to distinguish between the "able bodied poor" and the "non-able bodied poor", and so there was an incentive to start to separate the various categories of dependency and "deviancy" which had hitherto been lumped together. To continue providing aid to the able bodied would seriously undermine the emerging market economy.

People who were acutely disturbed did not fit well into any of the institutions then generally available: those who would not conform to workhouse rules presented a severe disruption; equally their presence in the local gaol would provoke complaint from both inmate and gaoler; general hospitals became increasingly reluctant to admit them.

At first the need for separate provision was largely met by a profitable private sector, paid by public funds to operate "madhouses", in which conditions were generally appalling.

A parallel, private profit orientated trade in lunacy was emerging, viewed by many as a sordid, disreputable business, albeit a highly lucrative one. The head of one, 'Brideswell', in Islington appositely named William Batty, died leaving an estate of £200,000.

There was, during this period, a new attitude to mental health developing among enlightened people. In the past madness had been thought of as possession by demons, and those experiencing it therefore had the status of animals rather than human beings. Now madness was seen by some as a human defect, which both demanded greater respect for mentally ill people and held out the possibility of improvement. It was thus that the campaign to provide public asylums as a better alternative to the workhouse or madhouse, gained ground.

"Lunacy reform" was one of the favourite causes of a plethora of distinguished philanthropists of the era, including evangelical reformers such as William Wilberforce, Lord Shaftesbury, Lord Robert Seymour and William Smith. The Benthamite intellectuals also rallied to the cause, including Samuel Whitbread and Bentham himself. A further force for change was found among local magistrates, who as the local government of the day, came face to face with the individual problems resulting from the changes taking place in society. They also had the duty of inspecting goals and workhouses, and so saw at first hand the conditions in which some people with mental illness were living.

The campaign to create asylums was not without its critics, and indeed there was considerable evidence that institutionalising people with mental health problems was not in their best interests.

County asylums were legitimised by parliament in 1828 and made obligatory in 1845. From the outset, the outcome was far from the rosy picture of a beneficial environment which the reformers had painted. The asylums filled up, and filled up fast, with people who did not necessarily have serious mental health problems. They included people found awkward or inconvenient for many reasons, people with tertiary syphilis, diabetes, lead poisoning, or simply malnutrition. A very high proportion stayed there until death, and the asylums quickly became seriously overcrowded. They were extended and duplicated, but as fast as more beds were provided, they were filled.

Tables 1 to 3 illustrate the developing picture of consistent increases in the scale of mental illness in the population and the corresponding increase in the number of people in the institutions.

This process was not without some encouragement from those in charge of the asylums.

It was a long standing belief, which they promoted vigorously, that the best chance of curing mental illness was afforded by early treatment. It was a common belief that their high rate of failure was therefore not the asylum's fault, but the fault of families who did not admit their relative quickly enough.

THE EMERGENCE OF PSYCHIATRY

Physicians and apothecaries had not had a great historical involvement in mental health, although "mad doctors" were one of the several groups who indulged in the disreputable but lucrative business of running private sector "mad houses". Their motives for doing so seem to have varied, but certainly among them was the desire to improve the lives of people they regarded as amenable to the treatments they had available. These consisted mainly of such things as purges, vomits and bleedings, and maybe coloured powders whose contents were a well guarded secret!

There were other views about the nature of madness and its treatment, notably the "moral treatment" methods pioneered by a layman, William Tuke, at the York Retreat. But medicine began to dominate the industry during the early nineteenth century, and with the growth of the asylums gained an unchallengeable monopoly.

Unfortunately the remedies they employed did not, of course, "cure" mental illness. What they did become proficient at was managing large numbers of people in an institutional environment, and their medical skills were of value when asylum patients had physical ailments.

In 1841 this new group of "experts" formed themselves into the Association of Medical Officers of Asylums and Hospitals for the Insane, and in 1853 commenced publication of their own periodical, the "Asylum Journal". Psychiatry had arrived as a profession, and increasingly became the personification of authority over the asylums, both within them and without.

In Western Europe in the 17th Century, the same imperatives produced similar response to the mentally ill, the institutionalisation of the deviant. The major difference particularly in France, being that the legitimisation of the institutions received Royal encouragement and resources and grew therefore earlier in size and numbers. From 1656 onwards with the establishment of the French 'Hopiteaux Generaux' started the great confinement and spread across other European countries. Thus the movement to establish a specialised institutional response to madness was a 17th and 18th Century phenomena in Western Europe and predominantly a 19th century one in England.

However, from the 19th century, this system of controlling the mentally ill spread throughout all countries of the world driven by a desire to create separateness from society, central control and market forces; the expanding Empire of Asylumdom! Until the 1950's this institutional response remained the dominant approach to the mentally ill, with a pattern of year by year increases in the number of inmates in the mental hospitals remaining unchanged until 1954. Since then we have witnessed a major departure from historical precedent, a reversal of the remorseless increase in the size of the mental hospitals. Even more abrupt has been the mental hospitals decline from official favour where many have now written them off as doomed institutions because of a mounting attack of their negative effects on those they serve.

Illustrated in Table 4 is a picture of the present situation in 4 countries. This shows the differences in the number of the beds in institutions in different countries in the world. Italy, England and Scotland have policies and Japan does not. Just relying on national policy isn't enough to make a move to community care.

A RETURN TO COMMUNITY CARE?

In the twilight of Asylumdom, since the nineteen fifties there has been an attempt to return to community care. This has been tried in a variety of ways:

Introducing new legislation to protect the rights of people with mental health problems. Many countries have mental health laws to do this. In Europe 24 countries have specific mental health legislation; Austria, Belgium, Denmark, England and Wales, Finland, France, Georgia, Germany, Greece, Ireland, Israel, Italy, Luxembourg, Malta, Monaco, Northern Ireland, Norway, Portugal, Russia, Scotland, Sweden, Switzerland, the Netherlands and Turkmenistan. Romania and Lithuania are waiting for their legislation to be enacted. Elsewhere in the world USA, Canada, New Zealand, Australia and Japan and many other countries have similar legislation. However, the practice of the law varies enormously. One recent example, that of Japan where the law is 4 years old demonstrated by the review tribunal system, which saw 110,000 people in institutions, reviewed their compulsion over a one year period and released one solitary person. The United Nations in 1991 passed a universal declaration to protect the rights of people with a mental illness.

National Mental Health Policy and Strategies. In 1975, the British Government adopted a policy for the development of locally-based, community health and social services as a better alternative to the traditional, specialist psychiatric hospitals. Other countries have adopted similar national policies based on developing services in the community. In the 1960's in the USA the community mental health centre movement was inspired by President Kennedy. In 1978 in Italy with the passing of Law 180 which prevented the admission of new patients to psychiatric hospitals (not the transfer of existing patients into the community) led the way to many centres of good community practice, Trieste, Prato and Verona. In Canada similar policy led to the establishment of the Greater Vancouver Mental Health Service. In Australia the Federal Government adopted a community mental health strategy in 1991 and in New Zealand in the 1980's national strategies were implemented to encourage the movement of services to community care.

In the UK in 1990's, some fifteen years on, progress in achieving the policy objective has, at best, been patchy. I know that because for two years I was attached to the Department of Health, touring the country to see what progress was being made in the mental health service, and I can tell you it was very patchy. Only a handful of districts have been able to devolve their services entirely and, in many districts, few steps have been taken towards providing accessible community services which reflect users' requirements.

There are many reasons for this. Firstly, there are few forces at work today that can compare with the forces that destroyed community care two hundred years ago. There are no reformers around today of the stature and influence of people like Wilberforce and Shaftesbury in the early nineteenth century.

Above all some of the economic imperatives which first forced mentally ill people from the community into the workhouse, and from there into the asylums, are still at work today, dragging back the movement to bring people out of those same asylums (for most of our large hospitals were built in that period). That force is the force that determines what, in the public sector, gets funded. Now, as then, there is no economic law which encourages the giving of help to people who, it is still widely believed, "won't help themselves".

Dr Rosen, from Sydney, has suggested that the de-institutionalisation of mental health services is happening more because of the expense of running psychiatric hospitals, and dissatisfaction with their deficiencies than a fundamental change in society's perception of the mentally ill. There is, therefore, room for some apprehension that once "long-stay patients" are resettled in the community, society may cease to recognise and fund them as members of "the deserving poor". This must not be allowed to happen.

COMMUNITY MENTAL HEALTH SERVICES

Over the last twenty years around the world innovative services have been developed by people committed and determined to introduce new services that will better meet the needs of people with mental health problems. These services have many common features:

a. Responsive to the needs and wants of the individual with a mental illness;

b. Local and therefore accessible;

c. One single point of referral and entry into the service;

d. Available 24 hrs a day, 7 days a week;

e. Providing outreach, attending to the users needs in whatever setting they may be living;

f. Ensuring continuity of care over long periods of time;

g. Integrating health, social care and support with housing, occupation, leisure and opportunities for adequate income and companionship;

h. Providing practical day to day support to meet the needs of users and carers;

i. A unitary financial and management system.

Community care is not, as some people seem to believe, any form of care outside hospital. Community care must be founded on the integration of hospital and community treatment and rehabilitation programmes. In the most successful examples, such as in Sydney

(Hoult et al 1984) and in Madison, Wisconsin (Stein & Test 1980) both the leadership and the financial arrangements are integrated, with money going with the patient from hospital to community to prevent it being used for other purposes. It is essential that our care management arrangements are fashioned in ways that will permit this to happen.

Community care must not just consist of isolated schemes, but must be a complete system, providing for a defined population and including a wide range of staffed and unstaffed residential facilities, in-patient and out-patient and day patient services, and outreach. It must ensure "early diagnosis, prompt treatment, continuity of care, social support and close liaison with other community services".

Some examples of these are:

In Madison, Wisconsin, in the United States, the Program for Assertive Community Treatment (PACT) approach provides both crisis treatment and continuity of care to small finite caseloads of people with enduring mental health problems. A small multidisciplinary team works in clients own homes, and works with them over an extended period. In a controlled comparison there has been clear evidence of PACT's more desirable outcomes and its cost effectiveness.

This kind of service has been replicated successfully in both large and small cities, including Montreal, Chicago and Baltimore, and in Sydney, Australia.

Sydney's Lower North Shore service has proved, by random a controlled trial (Hoult et al 1984) that people provided with comprehensive community treatment and a 24 hour crisis service are admitted to hospital less often, spend less time there, and do not prove a bigger burden on the carers. The community service achieved a clinically superior outcome and was preferred to hospital care both by those who used it and their relatives. It was also shown that these services cost no more than standard hospital care and after care. This service has now been in place for 13 years, whilst the Wisconsin, model which it emulates, is four years older still.

In another part of Sydney, the suburb of Ryde, there is a separate mobile crisis service providing treatment to people with a severe mental illness, in their homes, during acute phases of the illness, rather than admitting them to hospital. This has halved hospital admissions and greatly improved satisfaction with the service from its users and their families. It is important that results such as these are being achieved here and elsewhere in real life routine service settings, thus confirming the findings of earlier controlled trials.

In this country, at Sparkbrook in Birmingham (Dean et al 1992), it has been shown that it is possible to treat the majority of patients with acute psychiatric illness in their own homes. A twenty four hour on call home assessment service determines whether hospital admission is appropriate, or whether treatment can be delivered in the patients own home. A locally based mental health resource centre, an open referral system, and an active follow up policy add to the effectiveness of the service.

Also in this country randomised controlled trials in Southwark (Merson et al 1992) have shown that home care can reduce hospital stay by 80% and does not result in more admissions.

At Buckingham an approach has been developed (but not as far as I know formally evaluated as yet) which is fully integrated with the family practitioner services. It also combines intensive community mental health care with family and individual behavioural therapy. Other complementary approaches include a model of care in which families are helped to become expert in sharing in mental health care as part of a comprehensive package of care.

Other examples include: West Cornwall, West Birmingham, Gwynedd, Clywd, Stroud, North Lincs in the U.K. Auckland in New Zealand, Ottowa in Canada, Prato in Italy.

Critics of some of the results I have described have argued that the low admission rates achieved are because of home assessment or earlier intervention, rather than the twenty four hour availability of services. It may be that we need to conduct further research to establish precisely which features of the service produce the greatest effect. It is, however, unarguably the case that when all the ingredients of a comprehensive community service are present, whatever the precise mixture, the outcomes are better for service users.

THE EMERGENCE OF THE USER MOVEMENT

One of the common ingredients of the services I have described is a recognition that mental health professionals are not the only "experts" on mental illness and mental health. Service users and carers know a great deal about them too. Users can often contribute to finding their own solutions if they are enabled to make informed and realistic choices.

The user movement probably started in the USA with the birth of groups to protect the rights of many disadvantaged groups in society eg. black and ethnic groups, spreading into the area of mental health in the 1970's.

During the 1980s the mental health user movement in this country entered a new phase, with the birth of patients' councils (as in Nottingham), the extension of advocacy groups (as in Milton Keynes), the advent of national coordinating bodies (like MINDLINK Survivors Speak Out and UKAN) and the growth of a strong and articulate user voice. Through these forums people who use or have used services are beginning to influence the planning, management and monitoring of services.

Users in the Lambeth mental health forum have "forced the pace". They have instigated an entirely new planning mechanism, in which, every quarter, planners from the local health and social services departments meet in a summit with about 50 users, from every local mental health facility. In this case the statutory services appear to welcome the planning partnership and have put some resources into the forum's work. But the energy of users is not always matched by an equal commitment from statutory agencies, nor by a comprehensive planning framework.

Women have grouped together and set up women's therapy centres, in London,

Birmingham and Leeds, and a number of supportive projects like the White City project in London, and the Shanti project, both offering a combination of counselling and group support on deprived urban estates.

A National Advocacy Network has recently been founded (U.K.A.N), and the National Schizophrenia Fellowship (N.S.F.) now has many branches up and down the United Kingdom.

Some local services involve users on their management committees, involve them in running the service or have users on interview panels for staff. There is much progress still to be made but the highly significant process has been started of building services around what users want and need, rather than slotting them into existing - and often inappropriate - facilities.

Other countries elsewhere also have a strong and articulate user network for instance in New Zealand, throughout Europe with the European User Movement and in Mexico in 1991 the World Federation of Psychiatric Users with representations from over 50 countries was formed.

VOLUNTARY ORGANISATIONS

Voluntary organisations with special experience of mental health and mental illness should also be involved as partners in planning services. Their knowledge and understanding of local communities entitles them to be heard, and their contribution to planning and service provision entitles them to appropriate financial support.

In Italy a mental health self-help resource and research centre has been developed in Prato, to bring together people and organisations in the self-help movement. The intention is to form an umbrella organisation to permit the sharing of information, to improve the training of locality mental health professionals, to encourage mutual support with self-help organisations, and to establish resource files of self-help development internationally.

Seminars have been held involving users and carers, former users, voluntary and self-help organisations, and mental health professionals. The seminars are to identify and promote good working practice, and advise on methodology for specific research projects. It is also hoped to establish a European network of self-help organisations and to analyze specific situations requiring a self-help response in whole or in part, or requiring particular research projects with appropriate methodology.

WHAT WE NEED TO DO

It has been said that many committed professionals find themselves perpetually hamstrung, feeling unable to make sense of the system of care for their seriously mentally ill clients. Their time is wasted in futile efforts to pull it all together until they burn out or get out. This is rarely, if ever, their fault. The system is often in bits, pulling in contradictory directions, and might often be better described as an absurd non-system of care.

It is critically important that services are integrated, and Rosen has suggested that to be effective, integration of services within a catchment area must occur in at least two dimensions and on several levels: Services must be integrated over time - providing continuity through different phases of care, and integrated between different facets of care at any point in time.

The levels of integration are:

1. Unitary administrative fiscal and clinical management of catchment mental health services;

2. Acute treatment, rehabilitation, hospital and community care, by one service or team;

3. Case management bringing together all elements of service for and with individual service-users and their care givers.

4. Active involvement of and partnership between service providers, service-users, families and self-help groups;

5. Integration with local general health services, and close linkage to social services, housing organisations, welfare agencies and community groups.

6. Budget protection.

It is also necessary to harness what forces for change there are today. To harness these forces for development at all levels, internationally with exchange of ideas, information and people; nationally in terms of law, policy and strategy; locally in terms of creativity in service development by practitioners, users and carers, the voluntary and independent sectors. I believe that a collaboration of these forces is essential. Opportunities for implementing these lies also in organisational and fiscal change in market forces. If market forces forced the care of the mentally ill from the community to the institution in the nineteenth century, then it is arguably the case that market forces in the twentieth century can help in the establishment, once again, of community care. I believe that the two most important forces for change in the next twenty years will be the concept of purchasing health services, and the growing empowerment of users.

It is vital that purchasers, of both health and social care, are helped to gain expertise in the difficult area of assessing need and specifying services to meet those needs. It is purchasers who can control resources now, and with that goes an enormous responsibility to use them in the best interests of users of the service.

It is becoming increasingly well recognised that no-one is better placed to determine the best interests of service users than they themselves. With a little help from a few friends, or better still with some self-help, they can and will become increasingly able to define their needs and suggest how they may be met. Those of us who they communicate this to must be enabling too - we must learn how to listen. We have a considerable task to undertake together, if we are to overcome the absence of the dominant forces that took care away from the community two hundred years ago.

REFERENCES

Dean C, Phillips J, Gadd E.M, Joseph M, England S. A comprehensive community based service compared with a hospital based service for people with acute severe episodes of psychiatric illness. British Medical Journal 1992.

Hoult J, Rosen A, Reynolds I. Community orientated treatment compared to psychiatric hospital orientated treatment. Soc. Sci. Med. 1984; 18: 1005-1010.

Merson S, Tyrer P, Onyett S et al. Early intervention in psychiatric emergencies. Lancet 1992; 339: 1311-1314.

Rosen, A. Community psychiatric service: Will they endure? Current Opinion in Psychiatry. 1992. 5. 257-265.

Stein L.T, Test M.A. Alternative to mental hospital treatment, Conceptual model, treatment programme and clinical evaluation. Arch.Gen. Psych. 1980 37: 392-397.

TABLE 1

Number of Private and Pauper Lunatics, that Number Expressed as a Rate Per 10,000 of the General Population, and Pauper Lunatics as a Percentage of the Total Number of Lunatics

	Private		Pauper		Total Number of Lunatics	Pauper Lunatics as a Percentage of the Total Number of Lunatics
	Number	Rate/ 10,000	Number	Rate/ 10,000		
1844	4,072	2.47	16,821	10.21	20,893	80.5
1860	5,065	2.54	32,993	16.58	38,058	86.7
1865	5,790	2.74	40,160	18.99	45,950	87.4
1870	6,280	2.79	48,433	22.94	54,713	88.5
1875	7,340	3.09	56,403	23.55	63,743	88.5
1880	7,620	2.99	63,571	24.94	71,191	89.3
1885	7,751	2.82	71,215	25.89	78,966	90.2
1890	8,095	2.75	77,257	26.27	85,352	90.5

TABLE 2

Total Population, Total Admissions into All Asylums in the Year, and Admissions Expressed as a Rate per 10,000 of the Population of England and Wales, 1855-90

	Population Estimated for Middle of Year	Total Admissions Excluding Transfers	Rate of Admissions Per 10,000
1855	18,786,914	7,366	3.92
1860	19,902,713	9,512	4.77
1865	20,990,946	10,424	4.96
1870	22,501,316	10,219	4.54
1875	23,944,459	12,442	5.19
1880	25,480,161	13,240	5.19
1885	27,499,041	13,354	4.85
1890	29,407,649	16,197	5.51

TABLE 3

1 Jan	Population	Number Officially Identified as Insane	Rate Per 10,000	Source of Data on Number Insane
1807	9,960,000	2,248	2.26	House of Commons 1807
1819	11,106,000	6,000	5.40	Burrows 1820
1828	13,106,000	8,000	6.10	Halliday 1828
1829	13,370,000	16,500	12.34	Halliday 1829
1836	14,900,000	13,667	9.18	Parliamentary Return 1836
1844	16,480,000	20,893	12.66	Metropolitan Commissioners in Lunacy
1850		NOT AVAILABLE		
1855	18,786,914	30,993	16.49	Commissioners in Lunacy Annual Reports
1860	19,902,713	38,058	19.12	
1865	21,145,151	45,950	21.73	
1870	22,501,316	54,713	24.31	
1875	23,944,459	63,793	26.64	
1880	25,480,161	71,191	27.94	
1885	27,499,041	79,704	28.98	
1890	29,407,649	86,067	29.26	

1992 Statistics for 4 Countries

	Japan	Italy	Scotland	England
No. of Psychiatric Hospitals	1,663	-	28	1,000
No. of Psychiatric Beds	362,000	58,700	13,250	62,931
No. of In-patients	347,000	-	11,650	-
Psychiatric Beds per 10,000 Population	29.2	10.3	25.9	12.6

"EUROPEAN GOOD PRACTICE"

JOHN H. HENDERSON

INTRODUCTION

Twenty years ago, in 1972 Dr Tony May, Regional Officer for Mental Health in WHO Regional Office for Europe began to assemble the products of an extensive enquiry into comparative data made available by national governments on their services and resources provided for mentally ill patients "Mental Health Services in Europe"[1]. This seminal report, published in 1976, with a comparative analysis of available data and its evaluation of trends provided a valuable source of information and inspiration for many people.

Whilst undoubtedly the content of the report was largely retrospective, the real value it provided was not only in the descriptions of services and quantification of resources as published, but the perceptive forecast of things to come and the actions required to achieve improvement and development of mental health care in Europe in the future.

In the 1970's this compendium of data and prediction became a valuable reference and an equally valuable inspiration to many in health services' administration, in professional education and in political and public campaigning. All were well served by this innovative exercise of "Taking Stock".

Organisational models then, as now, could be easily classified as total state care, largely private care, or mixed private and state care. Within these structures of service provision the principal findings were of many and varied organisational patterns of local, regional and national services. Most of these revealed a near total dependence on mental hospitals as the locus of services. Throughout the countries of Europe, and within the countries themselves a wide variation prevailed in the provision of beds to the population being served.

Most revealed a near total lack of geriatric provision though some illustrated a development towards specialised or differentiated facilities in both in-patient and extra mural care, though alternatives to in-patient care were in general few and often confined only to out-patient provision.

The report revealed that although mental health care in Europe was diverse in many respects there was also much similarity. Each country in Europe had shared an asylum past, providing the mentally ill with at least a modicum of shelter and care, although the treatment provision was a significant variable. Many countries had shared the experience of the "medicalisation" of psychiatry current in the first half of the century and coming into relief (and question) in the second half of the century. This process of medicalisation comes once more into high profile in the 1990's and in some countries this issue today presents a major policy debate as to the appropriate locus for mental health care.

In many countries in Europe, after the Second World War, there came the advent of the "welfare state" or "socialised medicine". The report from May in 1976[1] gave evidence of diverse systems of national health and welfare provision some of which had many similarities but as is the case in national comparisons, there were also many differences. The period of May's enquiries in the early 1970's happened to coincide with the transition (significantly so in Western Europe) from the "affluent sixties" to the "economically stressed seventies".

POLICY INITIATIVES

At this point it is revealing and helpful to consider and remind ourselves of some of the major Policies which have impacted on mental health care in Europe in recent times.

1. From France in March 1960 came "L'esprit du Secteur" which consolidated by decree and subsequently by Ministry of Health Circular in March 1972 the principle of sectorisation encouraged further by a Law in July 1968 bringing psychiatric hospitals into general hospital provision and administration.

2. In 1962 from the U.S.A. came the blazing beacon of John F Kennedy's "Community Mental Health Centres" legislation.

3. From the UK in mid 1970's came the Ministry of Health policy statement "Better Services for the Mentally Ill" and its parallel policy statement for the Mentally Handicapped.

4. In Italy, conceived in 1978, came law 180 which literally, at a stroke, transformed care for the mentally ill in that country and profoundly influenced many others in Europe with its ban on mental hospital admissions and the mandatory provision of psychiatric beds in general hospitals.

However, not only were these nationally determined policies responsible for the trends of change, but also significant experiences of innovation and change of practice at local levels described by individuals. We need only to remind ourselves of Querido's pioneering community based treatment in Amsterdam in the 1930's, of Lambo's work in village communities in Nigeria in the 1950's and of the many pioneering initiatives of numerous charismatic and influential professional and public figures throughout Europe.

It was appropriate then that early in the 1980's WHO's European Office embarked again on another survey of mental health care in Europe. The report entitled "Mental Health Services in Europe - 10 Years On" was published by the Regional Office in 1984[2]. It was based on national enquiries and responses carried out in 1982 and 1983. This time, less dependent on the quantitative approach adopted by May[1] in his report, but enhanced with much more description of the characteristics of these services in use and being developed at that time.

For WHO the early years of the 1980's was an important time. Internally in the Organisation it marked the end of an era of long term development and resource support from the Organisation to many member states in Europe. It marked too a point of significant transition away from an international public health perspective of resource support for policies and their development at national level, thrusting the concept of Primary Health Care (Alma Ata Declaration[3]) into the developed and developing nations of Europe.

The WHO Mental Health enquiry "10 Years On" gave factual evidence of significant trends of change in methods of mental health care delivery and the structures used, frequently in response to changes in policies adopted by many countries in the period under review. This enquiry was greatly assisted by a WHO coordinated initiative which encouraged local centres of mental health care delivery to undertake self descriptive and self evaluation studies of their patterns and practices of treatment and care of the mentally ill patient. This unique mental health collaborative endeavour persisted for over 10 years and itself resulted in an important publication "Mental Health Services in Pilot Study Areas in Europe" published by the WHO Regional Office in 1986[4].

THE RESULTS OF CHANGE

Some of the (crude) indicators of change used to quantify and describe the trends of change in a number of countries included:

-        Reduction of the number of Mental Hospitals with more than 1000 beds

-        Increase in the number of General Hospital psychiatric units

-        Decrease in the length of in-patient stay

-        Reduction in the number of psychiatric beds per 1000 population

-        Reduction in the average size of Mental Hospitals

-        Increase in extra mural care

-        Increase in numbers of professional staff

-        Reduction in the proportion of compulsory admissions to hospitals

From the report itself the important principles of good practice of this era can be summed up as follows:

-        Continuity of care

-        Comprehensiveness of care

-        Multidisciplinary team approach

-        Development of alternatives to in-patient care

-        Ensuring data collection for monitoring and evaluation

-        Development of indicators and targets in the planning cycle.

You may agree with the optimism of this survey (or you may not) which suggested that the ever increasing investment of many (most) countries in short term acute treatment services was expected to reduce the need for long term care and that the increasing use of non institutional resources in community care would reduce or indeed replace the need for mental hospitals. The cautiously pessimistic finding of the study were that the needs of the chronically mentally ill patient and those elderly patients with mental illness continued to pose real problems for health planners, health administrators, clinical staff and the public at large.

The concluding optimistic note from the WHO's study was that Health for All by the year 2000 with its clamant call for accessible, responsive, equitable and affordable (mental) health services would be the produce of the decade leading to the year 2000. Underpinning and ensuring this would be the Alma Ata Declaration in support of Primary Health Care thereby ensuring good (mental) health promotion and community involvement in the care of the mentally ill.

A singularly significant event for mental health development took place in Sweden in 1985 at the Second Conference of European Health Ministers, convened by the Council of Europe, at which 21 countries were represented, where agreement was reached on a common strategy for mental health developments based on the principles of comprehensive community based services, for treatment, care and rehabilitation of the mentally ill together with a commitment to a programme for the prevention of mental disorders and the promotion of mental health. The challenge to the 21 countries has been, and remains in large part, how to translate policy to action, planning to implementation and how to find the proper balance of quantity and quality of service provision necessary to achieve these aims.

During the 1990's, in Europe, it has become apparent that there is a widespread dissatisfaction with the way patients are treated, not only in general medical care but also in psychiatric care. These criticisms are directed at mental health professionals themselves, their choice of methods of treatment and especially the social, psychological and physical side effects of current psychiatric practice. Stigmatisation of the mentally ill patients and their families remains a singular problem throughout Europe. Loss of self determination poses real challenges to consumers of services and their families. The consumer voice is rising and is increasingly being heard in many places though not yet in all. The current emphasis in this decade upon service delivery is now a qualitative one and no longer quantitative.

LEGISLATING FOR CHANGE

Given that this is an overview of Mental Health in Europe it would be remiss not to devote some time and to Mental Health Legislation as the ultimate process of formalizing the principles of good practice for the care of the mentally ill people. The significant laws relating to mental health in Europe date from 1838 in France, in many countries from the mid 19th Century and in some only from the beginning of the 20th Century. Some European countries have no legislation whatsoever for mental health. Many changes have taken place in existing laws contained in some of the original statutes which tended to promote only the cause of protection of the public and control of the patient.

Recent changes in the mental health legislation, certainly those adopted in the last two decades, have been designed more to prevent the need for compulsion of care and treatment, have increased the safeguards for confidentiality, patients rights, introduced appeals and review procedures and have promulgated stricter legal and time controls. Consent and rights relating to treatment figure predominantly in newer legislation, while some countries use the law to ensure the formalisation of changes in service provision and delivery. For example ensuring that mental health care is an essential component of general health care, making it possible for general hospitals to carry and conduct psychiatric provision, establishing alternatives for care in the community and in some, legislating for the abolition of mental hospitals!

One legislative and ethical issue persisted throughout the 1980's, and gained most notoriety in the case of the erstwhile USSR. This was the issue for the political abuses of psychiatry which gave great cause for concern worldwide and consumed the politics of the World Psychiatric Association during that decade. However, do let us remember that nowhere in the world is the practice of medicine let alone the specialty of psychiatry absolutely free from political and ideological influences. This is especially true for psychiatry however and the care of the mentally ill patient. Other states in Central and Eastern Europe have been exposed to charges of political abuse of psychiatry since the opening of the Iron Curtain. But others in the West also have had to face challenges and criticisms of their legal framework as well as their professional practices often with special focus on vulnerable groups such as mentally disordered offenders, children and adolescents and older people with mental illness.

This vexatious area of debate of good and bad, the rights and wrongs of practice continues to be an area of concern and becomes properly an important territory for the World Federation for Mental Health and its National Associations, which will given increasing attention to these and like matters.

AFTER DEINSTITUTIONALISATION

The policies, practices and legislation I have described have led to a process which has been encompassed in the neologism "deinstitutionalisation". One of the paramount and important processes within this movement is the provision of the ways and means of enhancing the social and vocational integration of mentally ill patients within the community. This requires that adequate and appropriate community structures as well as positive and prevalent community attitudes are established.

Social integration makes demands on accommodation provision, recreational and leisure provision while vocational provision demands that not only work opportunity is provided but also that work training is available.

Throughout Europe these challenges of adequate community provision to meet needs is encumbered and impeded at the present time by the added social burden of economic recession, unemployment and reducing levels of social welfare provision caused by the reducing GNP of all countries. Nevertheless, many initiatives have been taken and many innovative schemes of occupational therapy, vocational training and forms of sheltered workshop have been created and widely replicated in Europe.

Of current and increasing interest, given the fragile and uncertain state of the employment market in Europe, are those developments for the mentally ill patient in social firms and independent patient co-operatives.

Of course the Europe we know today in 1993 is very different from that of 10 years ago and the prospect of WHO european regional undertaking a further ten year review of mental health services in Europe is greatly to be welcomed. The fact is that at the last count there are now over 50 member countries of WHO Europe compared to the 32 of ten years ago. The new countries are in the main made up of those emerging from central and eastern Europe and from the independent states of the former USSR.

In addition we have to take account today of the influence of the European Community, (the E.C.) which, apart from the enormous social and economic development prospects it offers to its own membership, has also made resources available to those countries in Europe sharing its view on the need for technical development in terms of cooperation and collaboration. In consequence we have the means of incorporating countries such as Austria, Finland, Norway and Sweden in EC joint collaboration and concerted action projects in the areas of social affairs and social structures. In addition special programmes of aid support to the newly emerging countries and old members of the central and eastern european alliances as well as the independent states of USSR can benefit from EC programmes such as PHARE and TACIS which also envisage a role for inter-country collaboration.

Some of the issues emerging from the Europe we know today are the enormous disparity in finances made available in countries for mental health needs, the significant and everlasting lack of suitable data compounded by the current differences in meaning given to standard terms such as out-patient, day hospital and the like. While some countries control medical and health manpower reasonably well others display a great laxity of planning and of human resource distribution.

It was possible for his report of May in 1976 to distinguish fairly clearly that countries could be identified as one or other of the following systems of mental health delivery:

Private provision, State provision or Mixed provision,

the scene in Europe today is much more complex. The emergence of the voluntary or not for profit sector, small enterprises, cooperatives and far greater collaboration one with the other, is to be welcomed.

There is still a great deal to be achieved in the development of good mental health care throughout Europe and pre-eminent among the challenges are those old chestnuts of ignorance, stigma and sloth or lack of will to do what is necessary to achieve change. Here then is one of our greatest challenges for the remainder of this decade and I look forward to hearing from the meeting the messages of encouragement and example that I can carry through Europe as the Vice President for the European Region of the World Federation for Mental Health and the Chairman of the European Regional Council of the Federation.

REFERENCES

1. May,A.R. Mental Health Services in Europe. Geneva, World Health Organisation, 1976 (WHO Offset Publication No. 23).

2. Freeman, H.L., Fryers, T & Henderson, J.H. Mental Health Services in Europe: 10 Years On. Copenhagen, WHO Regional Office for Europe, 1986 (Public Health in Europe, no.25).

3. Targets for Health for All. Copenhagen, WHO Regional Office for Europe, revised 1990.

4. Giel, R. et al. Mental Health Services in Pilot Study Areas: report on a European Study. Copenhagen, WHO Regional Office for Europe, 1986.

Community Care - The USA Experience

RONALD DIAMOND

Scotland is at the beginning of a major change in the treatment of people with serious mental illness. The change in Scotland parallels a change that started several decades ago in the United States and people working in Scotland are in a position to learn from the United States' experience. It is important to understand both the mistakes made in the United States, as well as to learn what has worked well. It is commonly said that "those who do not know history are doomed to repeat it". In transforming the mental health system, it is important to use history so as to repeat the best parts of what has happened in other places and not the worst.

Mental Health: From institutionalization to deinstitutionalization

The modern history of organized treatment for people with psychiatric disabilities can be thought of as beginning with Tuke and Pinel. Hospitals based on principles of "moral treatment" were humane places that had relatively brief stays and reported excellent outcomes. Treatment was provided by staff who in many ways were similar to the patients, often sharing a common religious background and from a similar socioeconomic strata. These early hospitals were a revolutionary step forward in the treatment of people with psychiatric disability.

With these small, humane hospitals as a model, the various states in the United States began to build public hospitals. It was an exciting time to be involved in providing mental health services. These hospitals provided treatment for people who would otherwise have wandered homeless, been locked up by their families, or arrested and put in jails. They were a revolutionary step forward in the treatment of people with psychiatric disability. The initial reform movement attempted to develop small hospitals with few patients living in well-equipped surroundings. Unfortunately, these hospitals rapidly grew huge, became overcrowded, understaffed, and became imbued with a sense of hopelessness that people could never recover from mental illness. The number of people in state hospitals in the United States grew every year from about 1850 until the mid-1950s. Every year there were more people in state hospitals than the year before. By the time this explosion was over, what had begun as an attempt to provide moral treatment in pleasant places had changed into warehousing people under conditions that were too often physically terrible and dehumanizing. New patients came and few left, and finally the population peaked at 560,000 in 1955.

After 1955 the population in these hospitals began to drop. There were many reasons for this decrease. (1) There was the development of new anti-psychotic medications. While the new medications were undoubtedly an important factor, they were not the entire reason for the decrease in the hospital census. In fact, the population in state hospitals was beginning to drop even before anti-psychotic medication was in widespread use. (2) In addition to new medications, many new non-pharmacological treatment approaches were developed. In large part because of experiences during World War II and Korea, mental health professionals had become more interested in people with serious illness. Mental health clinicians serving in the military had found that many people who were seriously ill could recover if given appropriate treatment. (3) There was also an increase in the number of mental health professionals available in the community available to treat persons with psychiatric illness. At the end of World War II there were 3,000 psychiatrists in the United States. There are now over 30,000 psychiatrists. (4) An additional factor was the increasing recognition that psychiatric patients had civil rights. Courts in the United States ruled that a person could not be confined or otherwise deprived of liberty, even if they were psychotic or mentally ill, unless there was some overriding reason to do so. In general, this was interpreted to mean that persons with mental illness could only be hospitalized against their will if they were dangerous to themselves or others. Keeping patients in a hospital indefinitely just because they were mentally ill was no longer legally acceptable. (5) And finally, and perhaps most importantly, was the rising cost of hospitalization. Hospitalizations that cost a few dollars a day could be afforded. The increasing court ordered requirements to provide treatment, reasonable staffing ratios and reasonable accommodation meant that now in 1993 public hospitals cost two or three hundred dollars a day. Keeping large numbers of patients in a hospital could simply not be afforded, even apart from the legal and treatment issues.

State hospitals were initially a solution to the lack of treatment. Deinstitutionalization was a solution to the state hospitals. As H. L. Mencken said, "For every problem there is one solution which is simple, neat and wrong". Deinstitutionalization as commonly implemented is just this kind of solution—it is simple, neat, and wrong. During the 1970's when many of us began to seriously experiment with community based treatment, it was thought that the job was to get people out of the state hospitals. Actually, this can accomplished very easily. If the goal is to just empty hospitals, the hospitals can be bombed or burned to the ground, or one can simply lock the doors and not allow admissions. It is very easy to get people out of the hospitals The problem is what happens next?

Deinstitutionalization has two connected but separate parts. The first part is the transfer of patients out of the large institutions. The second part is to provide the appropriate treatment and support once patients arrive in the community so that the hospital is no longer needed. This latter problem of providing the appropriate treatment and support is the more difficult and important part of deinstitutionalization, and this is what is being discussed in Glasgow. Unfortunately, in the United States emptying the hospitals happened without providing community treatment and support. As a result, as all of you have heard, large numbers of people with mental illness end up in jails or homeless. One of the largest inpatient mental health facility in the United

States is now the Los Angeles County jail. This is not a failure of deinstitutionalization; this is the failure of providing adequate community support.

One mark of this failure to provide adequate community supports is the hospital readmission rates. While first admissions to state hospitals have stayed level, readmissions have increased dramatically resulting in what has been called the "revolving door". Patients are discharged because of shortage of beds, but readmitted over and over again because there is inadequate support for them in the community. This failure is not because of a lack of information about how to provide the necessary community supports. There is a large research base demonstrating what is required if people with serious psychiatric illness are to live stable lives in the community.

Research Findings in Community Based Treatment:

A large number of research studies have examined the effectiveness of providing community based treatment, and almost all of the studies have demonstrated that community based treatment is at least as effective, and often more effective, as traditional treatment that is more heavily based in the hospital (Kiesler, 1982). These findings are as robust as the findings on the effectiveness of anti-psychotic medication. Early research strategies examined the effect of discharging patients before the clinical staff felt that they were ready (Herz et. al 1979). These premature discharge studies found that the group of patients who were discharged early did just as well at follow-up as the group that were allowed to stay in the hospital as long as the staff felt hospitalization was needed. Pasamanic and his colleagues (1967) went a step further. His team provided a community alternative to patients already assessed as needing hospitalization. Patients coming to the hospital for admission were instead sent home with their family. The family was supported by a psychiatric nurse or social worker who visited the patient in the home. Even with few visits and minimal intervention, the patients sent home with their families did as well as patients who were hospitalized.

A number of these early studies demonstrated that patients could be discharged from the hospital much earlier than traditionally thought, and that selected patients previously felt to need hospitalization could be treated in the community. There was still little information about whether a community based approach applied to only a small percentage of the hospital admissions, or whether they were more generally applicable. The Dane County-based studies by Stein and Test (1980), now replicated in Australia, in London, and many parts of the United States, were designed to answer this question. The early studies took an unselected group of patients who were already assessed as needing state hospitalization. Only patients with a primary diagnosis of organic brain syndrome or drug/alcohol abuse were excluded. Patients were randomly assigned to a community-based, assertive treatment team available 7 days a week to provide mobile, community based treatment and support. The patients assigned to the control were hospitalized and then provided with traditional follow-up services.

The findings are overwhelmingly clear. The people treated with the assertive treatment team at home did better, functioned better, preferred it, and had fewer symptoms compared to control patients treated with more traditional approaches.

In several studies the assertive community based treatment has been found to cost less than traditional treatment; in other studies the cost is about the same but the new intensive community based treatment saved enough in reduced hospital costs to at least cover the additional cost of the community programme. The general findings from a whole range of different studies carried out in different continents with different providers, who have different ideologies, are all very similar. Almost all patients can be treated in the community if appropriate services are available. The community treatment results in less time in hospital both initially and on re-admission. Some clinicians expressed concern that avoiding a "needed" hospitalization would increase the risk of a future, longer hospitalization. In fact, the data showed exactly the opposite. Patients who were treated in the community were much less likely to be hospitalized in the future.

It is important to note that the positive effects from these programmes last only while the programmes are in effect. A year after the assertive community support is stopped, all differences between the experimental and control groups disappear. It now seems clear that people with a persistent illness need a persistent programme. Treatment needs to be less focused on episodic care, and more organized to provide continuous care for people with long-standing disability.

The issue of money is often given as a reason why these community support programmes cannot be developed. How can all of these new services be afforded? The real issue is not how much money is available to the mental health system, but how the money is being used. In 1987, Wisconsin which has one of the better mental health systems in the United States, spent $31.11 per capita on public mental health services. During this same period, Washington D.C. , which has one of the poorer mental health systems in the country, spent $128.61 per capita (Torrey et al 1990). Obviously many things cost more in Washington than Wisconsin, and the sociological problems are greater in Washington. Also there is obviously some relationship between the amount of money available and the quality of services. Clearly we in Wisconsin would have better services if we had more money to fund our mental health system. It is also clear that there needs to be enough money to make the system work—that below a certain amount of resources an effective system cannot operate. **The main problem, however, is not just about how much money is available, but how the money is spent.**

Requirements for an Effective Mental Health System

For two decades, Dane County Wisconsin has been developing new ways of organizing a mental health system (Stein et. al. 1990). Those elements of the Dane County system that seem most important have been independently set up in Sydney, modified and then implemented in Ohio, Connecticut, and Vermont. Systems of care in different parts of the United States and different countries around the world are likely to look very different from each other, based on context, politics, funding, and history. It now seems clear, however, that any system that is going to be effective, whether it exists in Scotland or London or Wisconsin, will have to be organized around some general principles that all effective systems seem to share.

There needs to be a clear priority of providing ongoing services to persons with the

most serious and persistent illness. No mental health system will have enough money to do everything well. It is critical, therefore, to decide on the priorities for the system. If priorities are not developed for people who are most ill, then clinicians will end up treating those people who are easiest or more verbal or more clearly articulate what they need. It is critically important to design a system right from the beginning that has a priority of providing services to people who have the most serious and most persistent illness, because those are the people who will otherwise get lost to the service.

The hospital and the community must be part of a single, integrated system of care. In a traditional treatment system with traditional funding, the hospital and community operate as separate systems. They might communicate with each other, they might refer patients back and forth , but they are controlled by different agencies; they have their own budgets, and they get into disputes about who should have more money. The community programmes have a defined pot of money and the state hospitals have a defined pot of money. In this kind of system, a community based clinician can hospitalize a patient, without the cost for this hospitalization having any impact on the clinician's program. Keeping that person in the community, however, might require that an extra nurse be hired, or that staff get paid for overtime, or that the primary clinician might need to put in extra time at the expense of time spent with other patients. Commonly, the administrators for the community based programs say that they cannot afford any of these "extra" services, even if their use would avoid the use of a much more expensive hospitalization. The staff in the hospital on the other hand, often find it difficult to discharge some patients because the community based programmes are resistant to assume responsibility for certain patients. The hospital staff feel that a particular patient is ready for discharge and should be the responsibility of community staff, and the community programmes often feel that they are too busy and not ready to accept the responsibility.

In Dane County we have simplified the situation enormously. All of the public money from state, federal and local sources goes into a single local authority which has all the money and all of the responsibility for both hospital as well as community based treatment (Stein and Ganser, 1983). As a result of this single funding stream, there is one system of care that includes both the hospital and the community. When a patient from the mental health centre is hospitalized, the human services board pays the bill for that hospitalization. When a hospitalization is avoided, that money remains with the board and is available for any services that the patient needs as an alternative to hospital admission. This might include money for a hotel room, down payment on a flat, hiring an extra nurse to visit the person at home over the weekend to make sure he is taking medication, or even hiring another service user to go and stay with the patient for a few days while the person is having a hard time. Money is available to pay for a hospital bed if that is needed, and local hospitals are very willing to provide a bed for a public patient since that is how they get paid. Alternatively, if the patient can be maintained in the community then the money also stays in the community to buy the necessary support services.

Figure 1

Funding Strategies

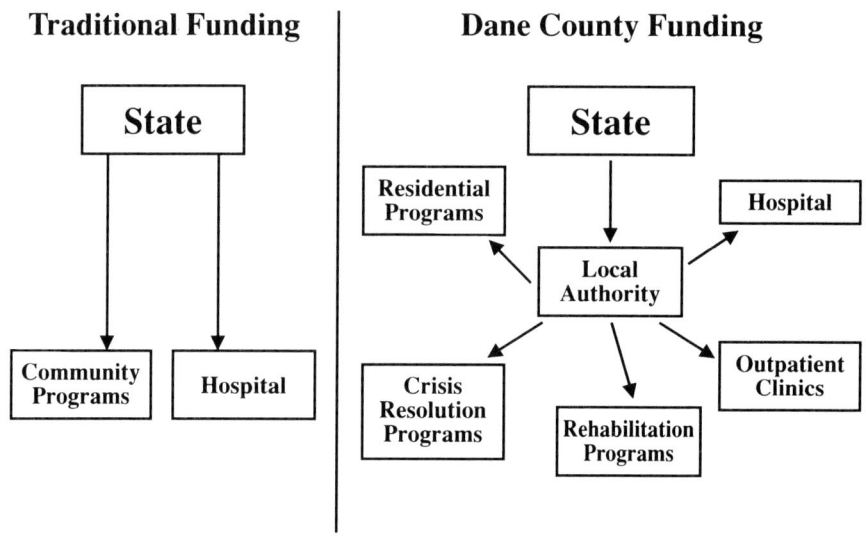

This only works if there is effective gate keeping to ensure that alternatives have been explored before hospital admission occurs. So far, this system applies only to public patients. In the United States, there is a split between private patients—those with money or private insurance, and public patients—those indigent or those already receiving services from the mental health centre. If a public patient comes into one of the hospital emergency rooms in Dane county requesting psychiatric hospital admission, be it at the nearby state hospital, the University Hospital, or a private hospital, the crisis team would be called.. The reason they would get a call is that the hospital would not get paid for the admission unless it is first authorized by the crisis team. That is a great inducement for the hospital to call the team before admitting a patient. Very often, the crisis team finds a variety of different alternatives to hospitalization.

Some time ago, one of my patients showed up at one of the local hospitals about 10 o'clock one night saying that the voices were getting worse and they were telling him to kill himself. The crisis team came over to the emergency room, sat down with the patient over a glass of milk and a couple of sandwiches, and discovered that he had spent all his money that month on marijuana, had no money, and that his friends had started avoiding him because he had been asking them for money and cigarettes and he had nothing to barter or trade in return. His whole world was beginning to collapse. He was stuck without money, without cigarettes, without friends. He did not need hospital admission – he needed help to re-establish his support system, to get some food, some cigarettes and some money to last until the next cheque came. He then needed help with budgeting his money to make sure this would not happen again. He did not end up in the hospital, but he did end up requiring services several times a day for the next couple of weeks as the crisis unit helped him to re-establish his life.

If someone does require hospital admission the crisis team will initially authorize two or three days of funding. After this initial inpatient assessment, the crisis staff, the hospital staff, and the client will all get together to come up with a treatment plan including the development of detailed goals for the hospital admission and an estimation of how long it is likely to take to meet those goals. At that point, the crisis staff may authorize another one or three or five days of hospitalization. Throughout the entire admission, the crisis team continues to have control over the authorisation of the payment for the hospital stay. The crisis team is not just acting as a fiscal agent, but also is directly involved in providing community based supports to facilitate discharge.

There were times when this entire system was new when an emergency room or a hospital was unwilling to discharge a patient and a confrontation would result. The crisis staff would come up with a community based plan and indicate that they were able and willing to assume responsibility for the patient's care. For example, the crisis staff might have assessed a patient and felt that their plan to see him several times a day in his own home, monitor medication, and make sure that he was eating would be enough to safely maintain him in the community. The hospital staff might respond that the patient was still psychotic and that they were not ready to release him. The crisis staff could not force the patient's discharge, but would indicate to the hospital physicians and administrators that there would be no payment for the period after they ceased to authorise the hospital admission. This kind of confrontation almost never happens now. Instead, it is a negotiation involving hospital staff, crisis staff and the patient. At the same time, it is a negotiation that leads to much more community based treatment because the community agency holds the purse strings.

Crisis services must be available in the community, 24 hours a day, seven days a week. One of the things found over and over again is that people get admitted to hospital at nights and weekends who would not have been admitted during the day. If patients are closely monitored, there will be fewer crises outside office hours. In Dane County we usually know if a patient has stopped taking his medication, is about to be evicted, whose mother is seriously ill, or whose girlfriend has broken up with him. We can often predict who is likely to have a crisis at 3 o'clock in the morning and it is less of a surprise when it happens. Even with this careful monitoring, we have found that we need to be able to work with a patient when the crisis occurs. We also need to be able to go out to where the crisis is occurring.

A few years ago one of the families with which I was working called to say that their adult daughter had locked herself in the bathroom for the last eight hours and was refusing to come out. This was a home with only one bathroom, things were becoming tense. Of course the traditional response was to tell the family to bring their daughter to the emergency room and we would then see what we can do. If

41

they could have done this, it would not have been a crisis. I remember going to the family home with some crisis staff and talking to the woman through the bathroom door. She said that she was in the bathroom taking a bath—we said we were going to start a family meeting in fifteen minutes. She said she did not have any clothes on—I said that I was a doctor and lack of clothes was not a major problem. She said the door was locked—and I said that I had permission from her father to break the door down in fifteen minutes. In exactly fifteen minutes she opened the door, fully clothed and we were able to proceed with a family session which included discussion about some very real issues she had with her parents. It would have been hard to respond to that crisis with traditional, hospital based or emergency room based services.

It is important for a crisis resolution service to have a range of alternatives available to decrease the need for hospitalization. People do get into difficulties and without concrete help things will often get worse. The Dane County Crisis service can pay for a hotel room for a patient who needs emergency housing, and we have been known to pay one service user to put up another user on their couch. A crisis home programme has been developed for patients who need a place to stay with other people around. We rent spare bedrooms from local families who have an extra room. We provide some training to these crisis home providers but the crisis staff provides the mental health treatment to the person in crisis. The home owners provide a family home that is secure and safe and nurturing, where people can go for a couple of nights if they just need a time-out from the world without resorting to hospitalization (Bennet, 1994). There are other times when patients can go back to their own home if staff are available to provide some extra support. This support might entail having the crisis staff taking a patient out for breakfast the next day, or talking to a patient's landlord about a threatened eviction, or visiting a patient's home and supervise the taking of medication if this is what is needed to help resolve the crisis. A range of resources and options are required to make a non-hospital community alternative to hospital admission effective.

Finally, we need to have information available 24-hours a day. In Dane County we have a central emergency telephone service which provides information. This information might include the patient's current treatment plan, what interventions have been effective when the person has been in crisis in the past, which family members or friends are useful in helping support the patient, whether the person has been dangerous previously or had other difficulties that need to be considered in dealing with the current crisis. It is extremely useful when working with a patient in crisis at 3 am to know that talking has helped to calm the person in the past, or that the patient has historically responded well to a particular medication, or even that the patient has never been dangerous in the past when they have presented in a similar way.

A clinician who is concerned about a patient can file a crisis alert with the emergency phone service, indicating the nature of the concern, the kind of crisis anticipated, what kinds of intervention are likely to be useful and what should be avoided. It is often much easier to be creative at 3 in the afternoon planning a response to a crisis with colleagues around, than responding to a crisis at 3 in the morning when you are working alone. It is useful in planning a response to a potential crisis to consider whether this patient is likely to be helped by a hospital admission or should hospital admission be avoided at all costs? If a crisis develops, should parents be involved or have they tended to inflame the situation in the past. At times, we work with patients when they are doing well to plan jointly how we can be most helpful if they have another crisis.

The mental health system needs to be organized around continuous rather than episodic care. Most traditional mental health services in the United States have planned most of their response around crisis stabilization—around episodic care. Most mental health systems have not been organized to provide the ongoing supports that will prevent the crisis in the first place. Too often, mental health services are time limited. Someone can live in a particular group home for a set number of months and then must move on, or can be in a vocational training program for a period of time but space must then be made for new people. This is very much like taking someone who is paraplegic, giving them a wheelchair, teaching them how to use public transportation in the wheelchair, live independently and even get a job using the wheelchair, and then after six months or a year taking the wheelchair away saying that we now needed it for someone else. We would never do this for someone with a physical disability, but we do this all of the time for persons with a psychiatric disability.

Financial incentives must be arranged to support good clinical practice. Part of this involves financial priorities. Most mental health systems, no matter how underfunded, have the resources to hospitalize a patient in crisis. These same systems do not have the resources to keep the same patient out of the hospital when they are doing better. There is enough money to put somebody in a hospital, which in the United States costs $300, $400, or $500 a day, but somehow most systems do not have the money to send a nurse out to make sure the patient is taking his or her medication on a Saturday morning, even when the nurse would be a lot less expensive than the hospital.

Until recently, about 70% of the public mental health dollar in most States of the United States has been spent on inpatient care. This percentage is now beginning to drop and the most recent figures that I could find indicated that 64% of the budget spent by states on mental health is now spent on inpatient care (Manderscheid and Sonnenschein, 1990). Until a few years ago 92% of the public mental health dollar spent in Washington, D.C. went to inpatient care. In Dane County we spend 20% of our public dollars on inpatient care which is how we can afford to have staff available seven days a week dropping off medication, taking people grocery shopping, helping them do their laundry, or supporting them when they start working by going onto the job site with them. Staff are available to sit with patients in a restaurant as they begin to re-establish contact with their family from whom they had been estranged, or teaching them the skills of taking a bus. We are able to do these things not because we have a lot of money, which we do not, but because we spend it where the patients are—in the community. We try to avoid spending it in hospital where most patients are not. That is how we can afford to do what we do and that is how we can afford to provide continuous care rather than episodic care.

Figure 2

U.S. State Mental Health Budgets: 1985

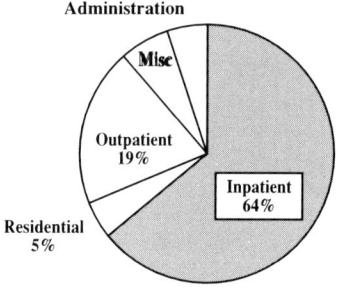

Figure 3

Dane County Mental Health Budget: 1992

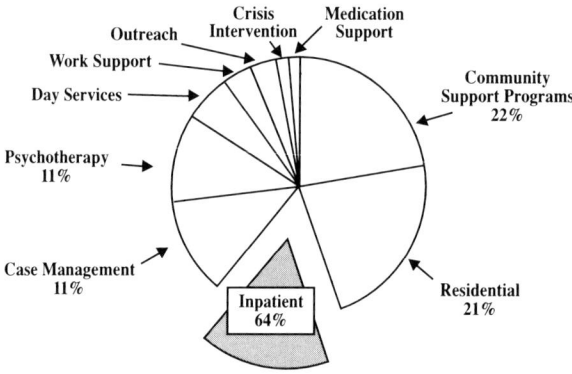

Figure 4

Hospital Use: 3 Years Before and After Starting Continuous Treatment Team   N=35

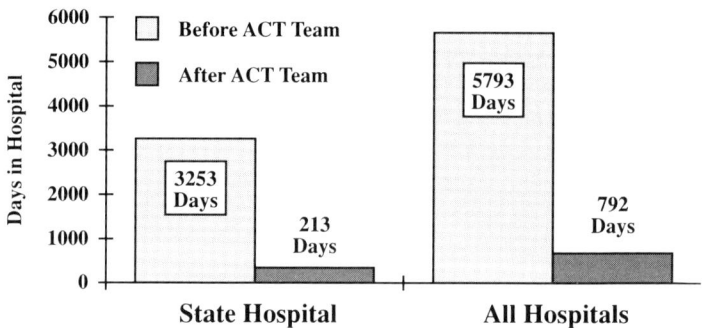

No matter how much money a service has as long as most of the money is going to the hospital there will not be enough money to provide adequate community based treatment. As a result of the system of care available in Dane County, the use of the state hospital has decreased from 5,600 patient days in 1977 when we started putting together our system of care, to a little over 1,000 patient days a year now (1993) for a community of 360,000 people. At any given time we have 3 or 4 people in the state hospital. We also have a county run long stay unit for the few people we are not able to maintain in the community. At this point we are running a long stay unit for about 7 people per 100,000 population. We have about 8 patients on that unit who have spent more than 2 years in the hospital out of our entire catchment area.

Figure (4) shows early data from one of our continuous treatment teams. We looked at the number of days patients spent in the hospital during the 3 years before entering the programme compared with the 3 years after entering the programme. Of the first 50 people in the programme, 35 were still actively involved with the programme 3 years later. This group of 35 people spent more than 3,200 days in the state hospital in the three years before entering the continuous treatment programme, and only a little in excess of 200 days in the state hospital in the three years after entering the programme. The total number of days in hospital is a more important indicator that just state hospital days, as the service uses the county and private hospitals. The use of all hospital beds for this group of 35 patients decreased from approximately 5,800 days to less than 800 days. This decrease in hospital bed use is the source of funding for the Dane County community mental health services.

The Dane County system has been doing what people are beginning to put together in Glasgow. The strategy in Glasgow includes the two cornerstones of an effective system- 24-hour a day, 7-day a week mobile crisis teams and effective case management. An effective case manager is not a broker of services who sits back in an office, but a clinician who is out there in the community, working alongside the client, making sure that things are really happening. An effective system requires a range of treatment and rehabilitation options.

We have become increasingly aware that if we are going to make community based treatment work, we need to ensure that our patients have real choices—choices about how they work with us, where they live, and how they spend time. Patients need choice about a whole variety of things that we used to choose for them. Patients need the same choices in life that we need. Personal choice becomes a very important part of keeping people stable and involved. It does not give a patient real choice to tell him that he can live anywhere he wants, but that no flats are available and only one group home has any vacancies. It does not give a patient a real choice if we tell him that he can get a job anywhere he wants, but there is only one sheltered workshop and there are no real supports to help him get a more independent job that fits more closely his own goals and aspirations.

A range of residential options is needed. Most of the patients with serious mental illness in Dane County now live in their own flats. We are following about 1,100 people who have a serious and persistent mental illness. Approximately 25 of these patients are in a long stay unit at the county hospital, 88 patients live in settings like group homes. Almost none of our patients live in nursing homes unless they have significant physical illness and physical disabilities. Some patients live with their parents but the vast majority live in their own apartments and homes. We find that most patients prefer to live in their own home and most can do so as long as specific services are provided to meet the needs of the patient that he cannot meet for himself.

For example, a patient might prefer to live alone, but is not going to be able to pay the rent without help. In this case, we have to make sure that we help to get the rent cheque out every month. Another patient might be fine about paying the rent, but be unable to go to a grocery store. If she does not go to a grocery store she does not have food in her home and so she starts eating in restaurants. As a result, she runs out of money early in the month because restaurants are expensive. Late in the month she has a crisis and come into the emergency room because she has run out of money. An intervention as simple as having staff go with the patient to the grocery store can allow the patient to learn, while helping to ensure that there is food in the home.

One of the patients I worked with had been arrested 77 times in the year before beginning to work with one of our assertive treatment teams . He was persona non grata in all the hospitals in town because he was so filthy and lice-ridden and unpleasant. The jail had left instructions that he was not to be arrested for anything short of a felony because they did not want to have to deal with him. He was very psychotic and quite paranoid. He was filthy and he looked strange and bizarre. As he walked down the street people would edge away from him and look at him strangely. When he got on a bus, people would give him lots of room. As a result of all of this, he becoming more and more convinced that people in the street and on the buses knew his entire mental history and that "they" must be broadcasting his state hospital records on the radio. The more paranoid he became, the more he looked at people strangely. The more strangely he behaved, the more people backed away, and the more he became convinced that "they" knew all about him. As this continued, he would become more dishevelled and look more strange and people would react even more strongly to his appearance. Finally he would start getting angry and end up doing something like breaking a window in one of the stores downtown as a way of trying to get back at the world.

Our intervention with him had many different elements, but one of the more effective things we did was that one of our male staff, about his own age, developed a relationship with him that he was willing to accept. This staff person would go to the patient's apartment (since the patient was unwilling to come to the clinic) and invite him to do things—go to a baseball game or to go bowling. The patient would respond that he was "not going to take any of that goddamn medication" but was willing to go out and socialise. Once the relationship had developed, the staff person began to suggest that the patient needed a shower before they went to the baseball game, or that the patient's clothes were filthy and that they should stop by a Laundromat and get them washed before the bowling. Over time, they developed a regular routine of getting cleaned up, going to the Laundromat and then doing something enjoyable, something social. After a further period of time, this developed into a good enough of a relationship that the patient was willing to try taking some medication. He has now been stable for several years and he has had no time in hospital or jail. He even started some classes at one of the local vocational colleges but so far has not been able to finish a semester. At least he has started towards his own goals in life.

This is an example of offering somebody a range of alternatives, meeting concrete needs and meeting them on the patient's own terms. Providing alternatives to hospital admission does not just mean closing the door of the hospital, it means meeting the patient's needs outside of the hospital. Often people need respite from the world or a place to stay, or help in dealing with a crisis. We need to be creative in making sure that there are a range of services available. If in fact we are trying to stabilize a patient on a medication and they need to be seen every day to monitor its effects, we can do that in the community. If somebody is too disorganized to take medication on their own and we need to make sure they are taking it twice a day, we can do that in the community. If somebody needs a place to stay that is quiet and that is away from their family or away from a room-mate, we can arrange that in the community. None of these are of necessity reasons for someone to be admitted to hospital. They are reasons why it is necessary for us to intervene in some creative way with some use of resources.

And finally, we need to make sure that the basic human needs of our patients are met. Providing mental health treatment, narrowly defined, is not enough to ensure community stability or a reasonable quality of life for persons with serious psychiatric disability. It is important for us to pay attention not only to things that are part of a traditional mental health service, but to the range of things that people need. When patients are put into long-stay hospitals, a lot more is provided than just mental health treatment. The hospital provides housing, a social structure, 24-hour crisis availability, medication monitoring, case management and integrated treatment. Many patients have some kind of job in the hospital, or at least daily activity that helps to provide structure to their lives. Other people are around, both patients and staff, providing some human contact on a regular basis. If we are going to provide alternatives to hospitalisation, we need to make sure that all of these needs are met.

Of all needs, in the United States a need for housing has been the most difficult to develop and has been the need most undervalued by the traditional mental health system. It would be very difficult for any of us to feel stable if we were living on the street. Providing a range of real housing alternatives is critical if we are serious about enabling people to live reasonable lives without the need to return to the hospital.

I have provided a brief overview about community treatment. I have tried to provide some information about mistakes we have made in the United States. I am sure that you have heard what we have done wrong - how we have made some bad mistakes in how we have closed hospitals in some parts of our country. You have probably heard how patients have been locked out of the hospital without other services being provided. There are

40,000 homeless people in New York City, and a significant number of those people have major mental health problems. This tragedy is not because we have closed the hospitals, it is because we have not provided the housing alternatives, case management and other services that people with psychiatric disability need to live stable lives in the community.

References

Bennett, R "Crisis Homes: Community Families as an Alternative to Short-term Hospitalization" unpublished manuscript available from author, 625 W. Washington Ave, Madison, Wisc 53703

Hertz, MI, Endicott J and Gibbon M "Brief hospitalization: two year follow-up" Arch Gen Psychiatry, 36, 701 (1979)

Kiesler, CA "Public and professional myths about mental hospitalization: an empirical reassessment of policy-related beliefs" Amer Psychologist, 37, 349-360, 1982

Manderscheid RW and Sonnenschein MA, Mental Health, United States, 1990. DHHS Publication No. (ADM)90-1708, U.S. Department of Health and Human Services Public Health Service

Pasamanick B., Scarpitti, FR and Dinitz S. Schizophrenics in the Community Appleton Century Crofts, New York (1967)

Stein, LI, Diamond RJ and Factor, RM "A system approach to the care of persons with schizophrenia" in Handbook of Schizophrenia vol 4 Psychosocial Treatment of Schizophrenia, M.I. Herz, S.J Keith and J.P. Docerty ed. Elsevier Science Publishers, 1990

Stein, LI and Ganser, LJ "Wisconsin's system for funding mental health services" New Dir Ment Health Serv., 18, 25. 1983 Jossey-Bass, San Francisco

Stein, LI and Test, MA "Alternatives to mental hospital treatment, I, Conceptual Model" Arch Gen Psychiat 37, 392, 1980

Torrey, EF, Erdman, K, Wolfe, SM and Flynn, SM Care of the Seriously Mentally Ill: A Rating of State Programs, A joint publication of Public Citizen Health Research Group and National Alliance for the Mentally Ill. third edition 1990

Acknowledgement

Much of my thinking has been profoundly influenced by Dr. Leonard Stein. Many of the ideas in this paper are his, and at this point it is impossible for me to separate out my thinking from his.

I want to express my appreciation to Marena C. Kehl whose careful reading helped immeasurably in improving the paper's clarity.

THE STRATEGIC PLAN FOR GLASGOW - THE TRUST'S VIEWPOINT

TIM DAVISON

Generating a strategic vision for a new community orientated mental health service which is shared and owned by all stakeholders is a crucial first step, but I would like to concentrate on how in Glasgow we are translating that strategic vision into service reality at the level of the individual service user. Successful implementation is the acid test of any strategic vision and the task is to translate glossy rhetoric into meaningful action.

There are six main areas which are central to the process of implementing the Mental Health Strategy in Greater Glasgow:

1. **Locality focus.** Greater Glasgow is a large, mainly urban, area with a population of almost one million people. It became quite clear that one single model of community based mental health services as an alternative to institutional forms of care could not be applied throughout the city in a rigidly uniform manner. The area comprises a number of communities with often widely differing characteristics including wide ranges in the levels of morbidity, mortality, deprivation and unemployment. The development of the new community based services is therefore focused on individual localities, with the model of service tailored to meet the specific needs of each locality. In this way, the new community mental health service in the east city centre locality includes a specialist team for the homeless which is not felt to be required, for example, in the Strathkelvin locality.

    For adult mental health services (16-65 years of age) we divided Greater Glasgow into 18 localities each with a population of around 50,000 people.

    For elderly mental health services (over 65 years) we used larger locality groupings of around 80-100,000 people; and for child and adolescent services we have based our implementation strategy on locality groupings of around 200,000 people. This paper will deal mainly with the development of adult mental health services in Greater Glasgow.

    During 1992/93 community mental health teams based in resource centres in the Clydebank, Maryhill and East City Centre localities were developed. This involved a financial investment of £1.5M in new contract income and £0.5M in capital investment.

The map of Greater Glasgow began to look like this:

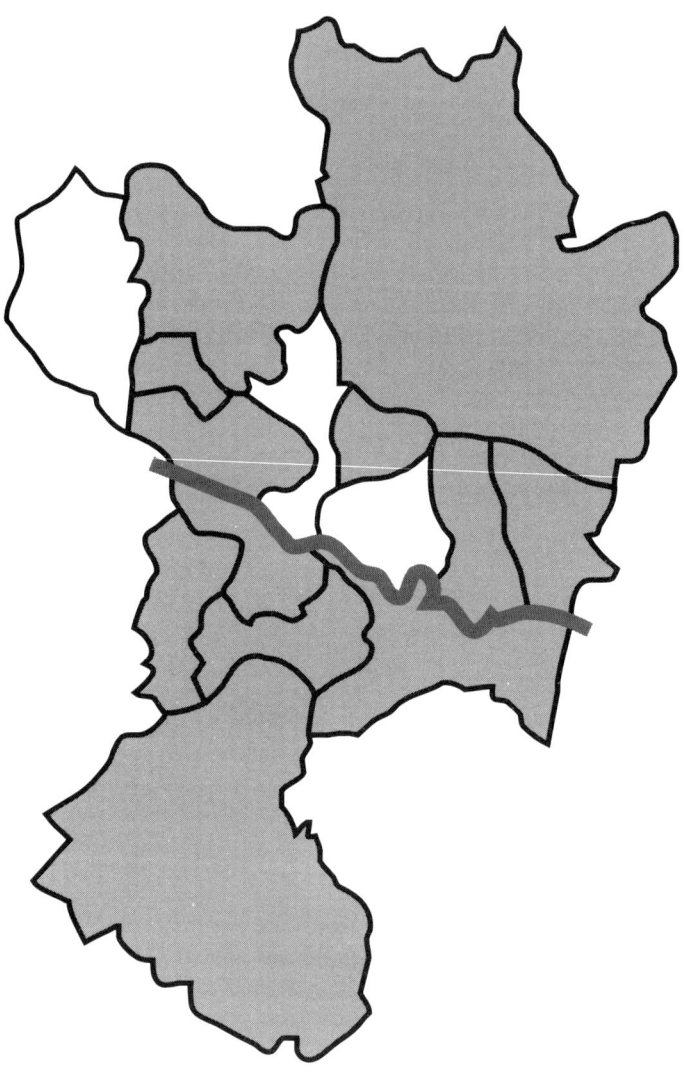

During 1993/94 three additional community mental health teams in the Strathkelvin, Easterhouse and Rutherglen/Cambuslang localities are being developed involving new contract income of £1.5M and capital investment of £1.5M. The map of Greater Glasgow currently looks like this:

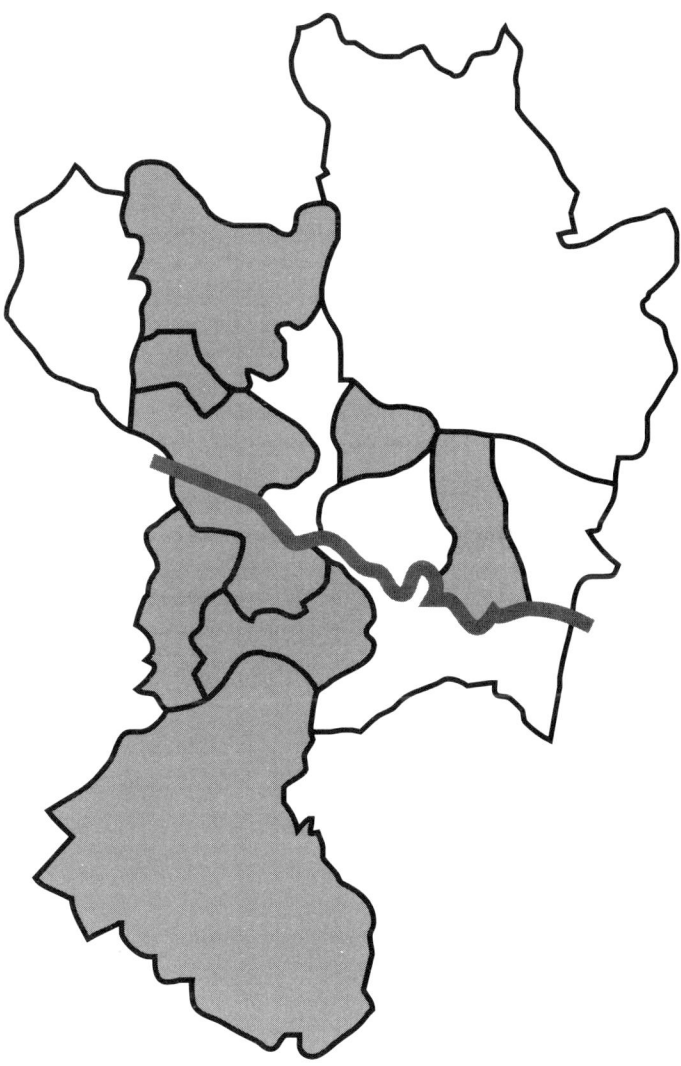

During 1994/95 we have firm agreement from our partners in the joint planning process and from the Management Executive of the NHS in Scotland to develop two further community mental health teams in the Springburn and Shettleston localities involving new contract income of £1M and capital investment of £1M. By the summer of 1994 the map of Greater Glasgow will look like this:

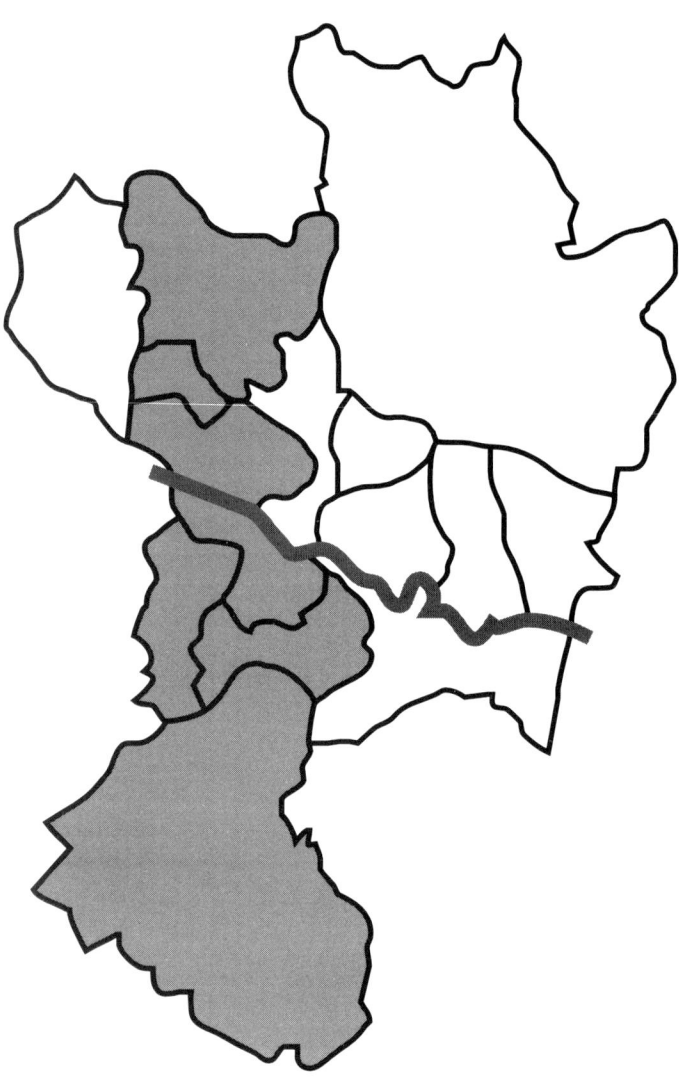

The scale and pace of this implementation should not be underestimated. In just 24 months, half of the population of Greater Glasgow will have been provided with well resourced community mental health teams providing services seven days a week, 365 days a year, with 24 hour on-call response facilities based in the community.

Of course it is not by accident that the new community mental health resources are concentrated around the North and East of the city as Map 3 illustrates. This is because we are focusing on the establishment of a robust community mental health infrastructure prior to the closure of Gartloch Hospital in the East Sector by 1995 and prior to the closure of Woodilee Hospital in the North Sector 12 months later. The key achievement from this process will be that the NHS community infrastructure will be in place at least one year before the closure of Gartloch Hospital and at least two years before the closure of Woodilee Hospital. This is in accordance with the central thesis of the Mental Health Strategy in Greater Glasgow which is to ensure that community services are in place prior to the closure of the institutions.

Locality Based Community Mental Health Centres. It is important to understand what the development of community mental health teams means for the delivery of services at the level of the individual service user. Before the development of the community mental health teams in the resource centres, each locality in Glasgow had a profile which looked something like this:

- three or four staff

- working Monday to Friday

- working from 9.00 am until 5.00 pm

- providing an outreach service to the psychiatric hospitals

In each of the localities with a developed community mental health team working from a resource centre the profile now looks more like this:

- over 20 staff

- working seven days per week, 365 days per year

- working from 9.00 am until 9.00 pm

- with 24 hour community psychiatric nurse (CPN) on call facilities

- where the service focus is the locality

- with access to sectorised beds which become an outreach for the community based service.

This fundamental shift in emphasis from a poorly resourced community service being a rather patchy outreach of a huge psychiatric institutional service to a system in which the robust, properly resourced community services become the focus of the service with access to a small number of in-patient beds when required is revolutionary, but it is happening. There is clearly a long way to go to ensure that the community teams work well in terms of internal relationships and, crucially, in terms of external relationships, particularly with users, carers, social work staff and general practitioners.

2. **Cash in, cash out, cash back** Everyone who works in the public sector is clear that resources are finite and that value for money is important. Hugely complex financial frameworks are now in place nationally to facilitate the change in the way mental health services are planned and delivered. The Greater Glasgow Strategy is based upon a sophisticated financial model supported by the Regional Council Social Work Department and the District Council's Housing Department through the joint planning process and supported by the Management Executive of the NHS in Scotland. Getting all of these agencies involved and agreeing to a financial framework over a five year period is an immense achievement which should not be underestimated and which followed the development of real synergy between the major purchaser and provider in the health sector. Long term bridging finance provides the 'cash in'. Long term cash releasing savings targets represent the 'cash out' and it is important to be realistic about how much money can actually be released from the institutions before they close. They have huge fixed costs and enormous capital charges and the costs of manpower reduction are real and significant, particularly within the in-patient nursing workforce. Even when the old buildings have been evacuated considerable resources can be spent securing them or demolishing them. As the residual patient population gets smaller the costs per patient are higher as the overheads of the large asylums remain largely unchanged. This clearly demonstrates the need for bridging finance until the institutions are closed but the institutions in Glasgow can release the cash which will make community care work in the city in the long term. It is important to be realistic about the pace at which that money will actually come out of the institutions and to recognise some of the real difficulties associated with releasing the resources tied up in fixed costs.

    The long term reinvestment in alternative community based services represents the 'cash back'. Although bridging finance is absolutely critical, long term reinvestment commitment from purchasers is even more crucial to ensure that the cash released from the institutions is actually reinvested in community based mental health services and that it stays there in the long term. One advantage of an asylum is that it is visible and everyone knows it needs resources. One of the disadvantages and weaknesses of community services is that they are very much less visible and are very easy to be disbanded or reduced.

3. **Capital and buildings** Mental health services are often referred to as being one of the priority services, and yet mental health is regarded in Scotland as a second priority to acute services for capital expenditure during the nineties. It is not possible to provide robust community mental health services out of tents and portacabins. There must be realistic, external financing limits and flexibility to buy, to lease, to extend, to upgrade, property or to go into partnerships with purchasers and other agencies in purchasing properties. General Practice financing of capital within Health Centres must be negotiated. There will be delays in disposing of

vacated institutions and significant losses on the disposal of assets and this must be taken into account. Effective community care services require space in locally accessible premises. As well as the rationalisation of acute services requiring a huge capital investment to allow resources to be released from acute services into community and primary care services a huge capital investment is also required in the community to sustain an effective community care infrastructure in suitable premises. There is little point in transferring revenue to provide staffing if the locations from which community staff are expected to work are cramped, overcrowded or non-existent.

4. **New services, new skills** New services need new skills. A very significant number of staff from the Glasgow institutions are being transferred into the resource centres but it is quite clear that 20 staff cannot be taken from a ward where they have worked for between five and twenty years, to a community like Clydebank or Easterhouse without retraining. New skills need to be acquired and this requires to be properly funded. Last year £100,000 was invested on training the first three community mental health teams in our first three resource centres. It is hoped that another £100,000 will be invested in 1993/4 in training for the next three teams, although securing funding for this crucial priority area has been exceptionally difficult. Training not only requires to be properly funded, it needs to be multi-disciplinary and multi-agency. Community care requires to be shared care. Shared care in the community involves a very wide range of disciplines and agencies to work together and it is clear that training needs to include all of these disciplines and agencies simultaneously. In practice this presents difficulties with overworked, busy people. Training is not just about skills, of course, it is also about attitudes and it is also about how referral agencies should actually use the new community based mental health services. Our staff need to be trained in working closely with general practitioners (GPs) and others, but GPs and social work staff also need training about who to refer to the community mental health service which is attempting to target people with serious mental illness so that the service is not overloaded with people with mild anxiety problems. There is a need for user involvement training and in the training of the first three teams, users were involved in telling the teams what they wanted from the new services and what their priorities were for service developments. Bridging finance is a potential source of funding training and Glasgow is hoping to use it in this way.

5. **Manpower reductions** Moving from institutional care to community care also involves the reduction in size of the NHS mental health services from being a monopoly provider of all, or most, mental health services to being one agency in a mixed economy of care working with a large range of partner agencies. The harsh reality of this is that the NHS mental health services require to shed jobs. In the overall mental health economy in Glasgow in the future there will probably be about as many jobs as there are now, but they will not be with the Trust and they will not be with the National Health Service. Four years ago there were almost 3,000 mental health nurses working in in-patient units. Now there are just under

2,200 and in five years time there will be something like 1,200. That is a huge reduction. In the last two years the Trust has invested £2M on a programme of early retirals and voluntary redundancies. Fourteen percent of the in-patient staff in Glasgow are on temporary contracts so that as wards close and savings are required manpower numbers can be reduced. Of course there is a danger that this policy will result in a loss of bright young people who are keen to work in community mental health services and a retention of some of the old guard who would rather go and that is why it is important to invest in early retiral and in voluntary redundancy to allow the new breed of mental health professionals in the NHS to come forward and to play a role in shaping and developing a new service. Redeploying and retraining of existing staff occurs wherever this is possible and all of the community resource centres in Glasgow involve redeployed staff who have come from the institutions. That brings with it another disadvantage in that we are not bringing in new blood from out with Glasgow. It is a disadvantage but it is required. The unit has also been following a policy of internal promotion which is a little insular and incestuous. However, it is necessary that manpower reductions are made in order to release cash to reinvest in alternative community services provided by these agencies.

6. **Pace of change** The pace of change is absolutely critical; too slow is as dangerous as too fast. The pace of change needs to be limited by the development of the community infrastructure and this is what is being implemented in Glasgow in advance of institutional closure. Coterminosity is an issue that we should be thinking about. The localities described earlier are not coterminous with social work district boundaries or even area team boundaries, nor are they coterminous with District Council Housing Authority boundaries. Local Government Reform is on its way and to wait would have resulted in delay. It was more important to ensure that the community mental health service was developed than it was to ensure that boundaries were identical. Once the resources are in place in the community, the boundaries can be renegotiated particularly when the shape of Local Government Reform is known.

Organisational capacity is of course an important issue. It is not just about the capacity of the Trust to down size and change, but it is also about the organisational capacity of every other partner agency, the private sector, the voluntary sector and social work services. The required expansion in the voluntary sector is of particular concern and must be supported. Patient and carer preparation is of course a clear pre-requisite for discharge from the institutions and people will not be discharged until the community infrastructure is there and until patients are prepared.

However, having said that the pace of change must be dependent upon these things, there is a great danger of going too slowly. The institutions in Glasgow and elsewhere in Scotland are slowly closing themselves as the elderly population declines naturally. The decline in the elderly population brings with it a decline in institutional resources. This 'cash out' of our mental health services in Scotland, and particularly in Glasgow, is inexorable. The Glasgow mental health services alone have lost something like £12M worth of income associated with the declining institutional services over the last four years. That declining in-patient income must be translated into community services and the pace of development must be linked to the pace of institutional decline. There is a huge danger that the institutions will decline and indecision about the way forward in the community will allow the money to run into the sand.

THE GREATER GLASGOW HEALTH BOARD'S PERSPECTIVE OF THE MENTAL HEALTH STRATEGY

ANDREW WEBSTER

The essence of this paper is a working example of collaboration between agencies and the flexibility and commitment required to maintain speedy progress. What I am going to do is to give you a flavour of the strategy which was approved by the Board in October. It's important to realise in developing a strategy we didn't start from a blank sheet of paper. So I shall explain a little about where we came from, then what is actually in the strategy in terms of its under-pinning principles and the key ideas and the needs which we have assessed it would meet. That will be followed by a description of how the strategy affects future services and how we plan to purchase those future services. I'll also cover the issues which have been raised with us by users, carers and other agencies because we have just been through a fairly extensive period of consultation both in the formal sense of the Health Board seeking written comments and also by talking with a lot of people within joint planning and users organisations in Glasgow about the implications of the strategy. Finally I'll explain the first phase of implementation.

In Glasgow we started from a very substantial record of hospital re-settlement and I would distinguish hospital re-settlement from community mental health services because I think they are two completely different things. What we had done was to substantially reduce the number of long-stay beds and over the past two and a half years, using bridging finance to establish the infrastructure of community accommodation and supporting services for over 200 people now living in the community; these are largely provided by voluntary organisations contracted to Greater Glasgow Health Board. Through that process the Board and the main health care providers developed a new sense of relationships with independent providers, not only with the voluntary sector but also with the private sector; long-stay patients with dementia have been placed with private nursing home providers as well as with the small-scale projects which the community voluntary organisations deliver.

In the process of separating purchasing and providing great strides have been made by the Community and Mental Health Unit in its business planning and as purchasers we were confronted with the need to keep in step with our providers. John Basson in his paper refers to a potential mismatch of talent and pace among purchasers and providers and it is important to be collaborative. There is competition between purchasers and providers but there was a great deal that we could learn from the work that had been done in developing the business plan for the Trust. We capitalised unashamedly on that because that was the right thing to do and I would encourage others to do likewise if they find themselves in similar circumstances.

So the Board found itself with a provider that had already articulated a vision with which it had considerable sympathy and wanted to build on and extend. In order to determine how much of the providers vision we wished to purchase we had to undertake our own assessment of need. Three factors have informed us on need.

These are imperfect insofar as information is limited, our capacity to interpret it could always be improved, and we need to forecast into a very uncertain future. But nevertheless it is important that we have as objective a basis for developing our ideas about future needs as we can get.

We took the epidemiological model developed by the Department of Health in England and applied the 'pyramid of need' or the 'iceberg of need' to the population in Glasgow. This suggests that, at any one time, of the 900,000 people we purchased healthcare for, 190,000 will have some kind of mental health problem, and of those about 160,000 will go to their G.P. Around half of those people will be diagnosed by their GP as having something in need of treatment. There is of course a big issue about the relationship between the GP and the patient and what is appropriately in need of treatment; this is something that our strategy doesn't address. Of those who require treatment 20,000 will access a specialist service as an outpatient and of those about 4,000 get admitted to hospital for a psychiatric condition every year. I've gone through those figures rather laboriously to demonstrate that the 4,000 people on whom we lavish immense attention are a tiny proportion of the people who actually use the service and that the emphasis which has been placed on shifting towards primary care, is not only founded on principle, it is founded on people's own experience of the service.

Having got that basic structure of need before us we then compared how Glasgow served those needs with comparable other places principally in England. I think the best example we used was Manchester and from this we concluded along with other evidence, that in Glasgow the service is inclined to treat people in hospital and to keep people in hospital more than almost anywhere else, in Scotland or in Britain.

This was borne out by the views that we received from users both in our own consultations as a purchasing organisation and at a range of stakeholder conferences which the Community and Mental Health Unit put together as part of a business planning exercise for the trust.

Unsurprisingly people wanted services that were there 24 hours a day, 7 days a week, were local, didn't over-react but did react when you wanted them. Now those sound very simple guidelines until you audit the existing service. Certainly, by hospitalising people, we frequently over-react and non hospital services are not there 24 hours a day 7 days a week. Those basic principles underline a more elaborate set of principles about how we want to go forward with mental health services.

The Board felt that it was crucial to establish a clear value base between purchaser, provider and the other agencies; social work, housing and voluntary organisations that are involved in mental health care, and there is within the strategy a set of common principles of equity, ordinary life choices, establishing that users have rights within the services and within the community which will meet some of the basic aspirations articulated to us in the needs assessment.

The second underlying principle is that we wanted to jointly plan and commission health and social care. People don't have health needs that go on forever or social care needs that go on forever. I find it, notwithstanding that it is my job to do so, very difficult to distinguish health and social care needs most of the time and I am convinced that we require services which can respond flexibly to health and social care needs. I also think that we should recognise that users simply don't understand the distinction between health and social care.

Thirdly, the Board was clear that we wanted to replace the Victorian asylums, not only because they represent a remote outmoded form of service, but also because almost all the resources we have to spend on mental health are locked up in them and if we want different services then we have to unlock these resources. We wanted to have comprehensive local community based services with a range of complementary providers. The Board is clear that the type of service which health service providers deliver will change radically over the next 5 to 10 years as will the services provided by private and voluntary organisations. My current feeling is that it is appreciated more by the health service providers than by others and that I think that there is a steep learning curve for some of the existing voluntary and private sector providers particularly providers of nursing homes and residential care.

By the year 2000 the following shift in the shape of Glasgow's mental health services is envisaged. At present there are 354 supported accommodation places in the community and including those people who will be placed in nursing home provision, that number will expand 4-fold over the next few years. Our day hospital infrastructure will expand from around 450 to 750. There are currently 4 community multi-disciplinary teams and it is envisaged those will increase to 25. On the basis of the investment in the community infrastructure, it is anticipated that the intensive care and acute beds will be rationalised onto small local sites. The issue of whether these will be on district general hospital sites has not been resolved and will continue to be reviewed during the implementation of the strategy; in the first phase in the east sector the acute beds will however remain in Parkhead Hospital which is not a district general hospital. The number of hospital continuing-care beds will be reduced from something over 1500 now to 360 by the year 2000 (see Table A).

What issues have people raised in response to the strategy?

- The first is the pace of change; are we actually able to implement this rate of change?

    Can we unlock resources from 2 large institutions (Gartloch Hospital and Woodilee

Hospitals) and invest it in comprehensive community infrastructure in the next 3-4 years? We have to if that degree of change is going to be achieved. It has to be done over a relatively short space of time not only on economic grounds but also in terms of establishing credible alternative services. The community infrastructure has to be seen to be 'the service' early in this process, not late. So we plan to invest heavily and quickly in the community infrastructure to show that that is where our purchasing priorities and our purchasing effort will go.

- The second question which is raised by people in the discussions is can we afford the strategy? The strategy sets out exactly what the Board spends now on mental health and what we envisage the replacement service will cost. This shows that within the total envelope of resources we currently commit the replacement service is affordable. There will be the costs of change on the way which the Board is seeking to support with bridging finance, but at the end of the day we are confident that we can afford the service we want. The Board has broken down the total spend by sector and hospital so we are achieving 'transparency' by sharing that data with our colleagues from social work and housing and inviting them to put the resources that they can commit to the future of mental health services on the table as well. When planning the replacement services for each sector we see the totality of the service across all agencies and the totality of funding available to purchase the services and that is the basis on which we determine allocations and purchasing priorities year on year.

- The third issue which has been raised particularly by general practitioners (G.P's) is our expectations of G.P.'s in this process and how will our links with them work so that a real emphasis on primary care can be delivered. The Board is very clear that it sees an increased role for general practice and for primary care as a whole in the delivery of these services. We are anxious that, essentially technical questions about the control of resources through fund-holding, attached staff, distribution of community nursing staff, will not cloud the essential question about the purchasing partnership between general practitioners as a whole in Glasgow and the Board in delivering strategic change. The Board has a lot to do in working with the general practitioners both through the facilitators that we currently have helping us with purchasing and with wider G.P. networks in achieving a shift to primary care in the delivery of mental health services.

Briefly what are we going to do next, now that we have this vision endorsed and these plans in place? Well we're already doing the detailed planning of the first phase of implementing this strategy which is a comprehensive service for the East sector of Glasgow. We are embarking on the planning of the second phase which involves services in the North sector. We have in place multi-disciplinary assessment of the existing patients in Gartloch Hospital. We have a programme of replacement services in terms of community teams, supported accommodation, nursing home placements, respite care, carer support, home support for people with mental illness, social work participation in the multi-disciplinary teams. We have identified year by year through the programme the hospital resources that can be released and their likely destination. We have established a joint commissioning team which has representatives from the social work department and the housing department, the provider and the purchaser and has an accountability to a joint planning group comprising the senior officers of all those agencies.

We have to secure bridging finance for at least three years to deliver this programme.

If you do the full programme planning that we have done then you have to get commitment to delivering it over a long period. I think we've gone a long way to securing real commitment in Glasgow and I hope that, given not only a fair wind in terms of resources, but a fair wind in continuing good relationships between purchaser and provider and the other key agencies we will have a model of how it is possible to achieve a radical shift in a short space of time.

A Vision of Future Services

- from 354 to 1275 community supported accommodation and nursing home places

- from 462 to 755 day hospital places

- from 4 to 25 multi-disciplinary teams

- from 52 to 45 intensive care beds

- from 1575 to 360 hospital continuing care beds

THE STRATEGIC PLAN FOR GLASGOW - THE SOCIAL SERVICES VIEWPOINT

MARY C. HARTNOLL

"Joint undertakings stand a better chance when they benefit both sides."

You might think that was a quote from the latest circular from the NHS Management Executive - though perhaps circulars are not usually quite so elegant. It is in fact a quote from Euripedes from 400 B.C. I wonder what experience had led him to make the comment.

Establishing a joint strategy in Scotland for establishing new community based services and for closing large outdated mental hospitals has taken us a long time. It is 30 years since the policy was first announced in England by David Ennals. When I came to work in Scotland 16 years ago, I joined the Programme Planning Group which was set up in 1975 by the Scottish Health Service Planning Council and the Advisory Council on Social Work. It took 10 years to produce its report 'Mental Health in Focus'. By that time the Advisory Council on Social Work had long since disappeared. The report cautiously recommended both the retention of a major role for hospitals and an increased community based mental health service. The problem was not in the document itself but in the absence of any change in direction at a national level. This meant that there was continued investment of capital in hospital building, a continued increase in revenue spending by the Department of Social Services on residential and nursing home care and the continued minimum expenditure by local authorities in respect of mental health - unlike spending on people with learning difficulties which expanded dramatically in response to pressure from families who had looked after their children at home and who rightly expected services when they reached school leaving age. Sadly, the stigma attached to mental illness has always meant that families are less vocal in demanding services. The lack of public sympathy meant that there were very few voluntary bodies active in the field. The most active a few years ago were those campaigning for the rights of mentally ill people in relation to compulsory admission rather than the need to develop services.

The absence of a national strategy did not mean that nothing at all happened. The hospitals did not close but there was a steady reduction in the number of adults with a mental illness accommodated in them. The problem was that some of their places were taken by the elderly with dementia and no resources were transferred to the community to allow mentally disordered people to be given the care they needed. As a consequence, many more people with a mental disorder became homeless and the number of mentally disordered offenders sentenced to imprisonment increased. At the time of the Planning Group the Scottish Prison Service met with us and said there was no significant problem of offenders with a mental disorder being sent to prison inappropriately. The report does make mention of the increasing incidence of drug abuse problems and the need for support for some remand prisoners. The position today is significantly different.

In short, therefore, the absence of a national strategy gave care in the community a bad name even before we had begun to plan for implementation of the actual legislation and long before the formal transfer of responsibility in April this year.

Over the past 3 years there has been a fundamental change both nationally and locally. We are now grappling jointly with the real issues involved. We recognise that there will not be public money available both for a large hospital sector **and** a community based service. We agree that confused elderly people should not be admitted to institutional care if they can be looked after in a smaller setting near their relatives and friends. We agree that people who are no longer ill should not stay long term in hospital but should be offered rehabilitation and support in the community. We agree we need to close the institutions and transfer resources to the community. How are we going to achieve it?

The process has already started but we have a long way to go. Greater Glasgow Health Board spends something like £80m on hospital services for the mentally ill and social work spends something like £4m in Glasgow. The recent availability of the Mental Illness Specific Grant has allowed some home support and day services to develop.

Bridging finance has facilitated the discharge of some patients and has allowed the financial planning of the transfer to proceed with some confidence. We have agreed that the shift in the balance of service provision away from the hospital and towards the community will require a major transfer of resources from health to social work. The nature of mental illness requires a high level of investment in health services in the community so that there are effective services available 24 hours a day. A joint approach is needed but within that, there must be as much clarity as possible about who provides which services.

We have made progress on identifying need. Glasgow has the highest admission rate and largest number of long stay residents per head of the population in Scotland, even allowing for the level of deprivation in the city. Consultation has established a shared view amongst consumers and professionals that there is a lack of community alternatives to hospital admission.

On an individual basis, a standardised assessment tool is being used in the programme for the closure of Gartloch hospital. This ensures both a joint professional approach and the involvement of users and carers in a structured way.

We have established the main elements of the service we want to see by the end of the century and perhaps more importantly, we have done so on the basis of firm assumptions about resources. The programme is optimistic in timescale but not unrealistic. There will be continued social work input to the short term hospital units and to the reducing hospital provision for continuing care. There will be social work input to the multi-disciplinary teams working on a specialist basis in localities across the city.

Supported accommodation in the community will be developed following joint agreement on the service needed although the contracting element will be undertaken by social work with resource transfer. The assessment of need so far has identified a requirement for 4 main levels of supported accommodation. The **first** would cater for frail, highly dependent patients many of whom are elderly. They will require 24 hour nursing support and typically this would be provided in a nursing home. The **second** level would be where staff need to be available on a 24 hour basis though not necessarily on waking duty. Continuous nursing would not be required and the size of units might vary between about 6 and 15 places. The **third** level of medium dependency would provide daily but not continuous support care and cluster projects might offer the most flexible form of accommodation. The **fourth,** low dependency group would be as far as possible in ordinary housing with planned support. The number of places required in Glasgow would increase from the current level of 350 places to nearly 1300 by the year 2000. Most of these places will be purchased from the independent sector. The demands for housing are obviously considerable and the need for capital investment may limit which agencies can participate.

There is a real problem over time scales to consult with users, with other agencies and to agree on projects and then to identify location, consult with local people and staff. The lead- in time is considerable but the problem of capital is real. The NHS capital programme is itself a very slow process. Small projects are being held back because of problems of capital.

Training has been mentioned. There is already a shortage of social workers and occupational therapists. Many with nursing qualifications will move to community but that will not be the choice of many. We need to develop a personnel strategy to deliver the service we all wish to see.

Home care services are already being developed locally and these will need to develop further, together with day and respite services. The need of carers for support and services has been identified as an essential part of the strategy. Employment and occupation schemes that re-establish confidence are beginning to develop although much more needs to be done.

The social work department is responsible for assessment and care management in respect of the social care needs of individuals. Some say that care management is not new. But what we are trying to achieve is fundamentally different from what has been offered in the past. The starting point is not 'Do you need the services we have on offer' - or in other words, assessing someone to see whether their need fits what we can provide. The emphasis is rather on what the individual needs and then trying to devise a service which meets those assessed needs. There will still be budget constraints and we will not be able to meet all needs - but we must ensure that a needs led service influences the kind of services that are developed.

In assessing social care need in the context of people with a mental illness, the care manager will be working as part of a multi-disciplinary team in the specialist service. The care plan will be part of a wider plan to ensure the health and social care needs of the individual are met.

Care management for elderly people will be part of the service offered from area teams. A key responsibility of the community care teams in social work is to work with general practitioners (GPs). It is estimated that 30% of people currently referred to area teams have a significant mental health element to their problems although they are rarely described in those terms. Similarly referrals to the GP often include an underlying problem of mental health. Community care teams in social work will continue to provide a generic service to people with mental health problems. Discussion is going on about the extent of the need for services for people with dementia to be specialist. We anticipate at this stage that the assessment and care management of people with dementia who are currently in the community will be provided for the community care teams but that some of the services to be developed will be specialist. The programme to replace hospital places for people with dementia will require a specific input of staff for assessment and care management. As far as possible though, the emphasis will not be on moving people out of hospital unless they can be better cared for elsewhere. We need to develop alternatives so that new admissions are no longer needed. This will require input to the commissioning process based on a more general assessment of need.

So, by the end of the century, we hope to see

- a much smaller but modern hospital service providing mostly short term and crisis intervention but also a continued provision of forensic units and some continuing care beds for people who could not be discharged.

- comprehensive access to community based multi-disciplinary services.

- a range of residential options from nursing homes to supported tenancies.

- home care, day care, respite and employment services.

There are two further threads which must run through our services. People with a mental illness are vulnerable. Our experience in all settings is that vulnerable people who receive poor services do not complain - or if they do, they are not heard. If the changes we are making are to be truly radical, we must achieve a shift in power to the user of services. The best way of building this into the system is to ensure the needs assessment at the individual level gives real power to the consumer to choose the service he or she would prefer - and to ensure that there are effective advocacy services that are independent of service providers.

The second thread is the issue of public confidence. We cannot avoid all risk but there is a tremendous fear of mental illness which is unleashed at the slightest incident. The majority of people to be accommodation in the community are probably elderly and no risk at all to others. We need to provide the best information to the public that we can about the processes and safeguards in the systems whilst maintaining confidentiality for the individual. Community care does not change the procedures in respect of people who are known to be a risk to the public.

And so finally, any plan must be reviewed. We must take less time to implement the strategy than it did to formulate it. But we must adapt it as we proceed. As Sir Edmund Burke said in 1977 in a letter to the Sheriffs of Bristol:

"Nothing in Progression can rest on its original plan."

PREPARING THE PROFESSIONS FOR COMMUNITY CARE - PSYCHIATRISTS

PROFESSOR CHRIS THOMPSON

In considering the training or preparation of the medical and other professions for community care, it is better to think of a comprehensive service rather than a purely "community" service. Any major shift in the orientation of services from institutional based services to community based services is bound to need a period of re-training, or at least of re-orientation. I'd like to discuss three aspects of training.

First, we need to make sure that our professionals are training in the right way in training schemes of high quality in terms of their teaching methodology and their clinical orientation. They should be trained to deliver quality services, in terms of formal quality standards, access to services, user satisfaction and so on.

But there's another factor and that is training the right <u>number</u> of professionals to provide an adequate community care service. There's very little doubt that community care requires a greater number of professionals to deliver the service than old style institutional care did. Statements such as: "Provider projections of the number of qualified nurses required for the new services indicate a significant reduction over the next five years by comparison with existing levels." (Water Tower 1993, DOH) are entirely opposed to the view that I would have: that you need more professionals to provide an adequate community care service than an institutionalised service.

The numbers of trainees in the medical profession, for psychiatry and other secondary care services are controlled (in England by the Joint Planning Advisory Committee, and in Scotland by a similar organisation) and that restricts the number of doctors who can become consultants. Although that approach evens out the pyramid for medical careers, it does deliberately lead to restrictions on the number of available trained staff. The numbers in psychiatry are constantly being reviewed and revised upwards in many cases but there is an inevitable lag period before they are available as fully trained specialists. Furthermore many trusts are reluctant to pay for trainees allocated to their regions, further reducing the numbers of trained staff.

When reviewing community care systems operating in the United States which may be under consideration for this country it's important to be aware that in the UK we have 3.5 psychiatrists per hundred thousand population compared with 13.6 in the United States. Community care is only possible with the right number of staff, trained in the right way.

The Royal College of Psychiatrists, for about twenty years, has had a system of approval visits to training schemes. These occur at least once every five years and there has been a gradual amalgamation of training posts over that time into bigger and bigger schemes, in order to widen the amount of experience that individual trainees can access. This therefore regulates the quality and variety of the training to which individual trainees are exposed. At the visits to the scheme the College visitors look for good quality clinical supervision by a consultant - so the "apprenticeship model" is in the forefront of their minds. The adequacy of the training environment is also important. The College wants to be sure that psychiatric trainees are training in good quality services and getting a good experience of that service. Obviously that can only be done as services develop high quality standards. It was difficult, in the early years of this exercise to make sure that trainees did get a good training experience, but as community services begin to develop so more training places become available in the community and College visitors actively encourage their incorporation into training schemes.

Another aspect which is examined at these approval visits is the quality of information services, e.g. libraries. Psychotherapy is taken very seriously as an element of training, and that would includes counselling skills, communication skills and interview skills. The College also insists that a training in various forms of psychotherapy should be mandatory for psychiatric trainees. Last but not least, there must be evidence that multidisciplinary teams are working well and that trainees are getting experience of working in them. If there are deficiencies in enough of these and other aspects of training the College can and does remove its approval for training from the scheme which means that new trainees cannot be recruited unless and until the deficiencies are rectified. This is a powerful tool in raising standards.

These training schemes go on for about three years of the trainee's life after registration as a doctor and very often after previous experience in general practice or general medicine. The most commonly reported problem with them is that trainees tend to rotate quite rapidly, every six to nine months and so their experience of continuing of care, of looking after people over a long period of time, is delayed until later in their training. Trainees usually gain experience in old age psychiatry as well as general psychiatry, child and adolescent psychiatry, forensic psychiatry and psychotherapy, some also gain experience in the psychiatry of learning disabilities, some in substance misuse and some in other areas of medicine such as general practice. In addition to that they have a three year day release course of academic training in social and psychological as well as biomedical aspects of psychiatry.

Once a trainee has obtained their membership of the Royal College of Psychiatrists they then go on to do senior registrar training in the specialty in which they are hoping to gain a consultant post.

Let us examine which are the essential elements for training psychiatrists to work in the community. The content of the training would be same; basic clinical skills like communication skills, interview skills, discussing treatment plans with patients, and so on are as important to community services as to in-patient services. The need for basic education in psychiatry and psychopathology - (by that I mean understands the experience that the patient is having and trying to formulate their experience in order to come to a treatment plan) is also important. A solid grounding in the knowledge - base of the discipline is important and this must be based on research findings including health services research. The trainee must be taught how to understand the results of published research. This latter helps all professions to avoid dogma which is so prevalent in mental health services and, more importantly perhaps, to know what is unknown - to know where the limits of knowledge lie so that the trainee can be modest but realistic in their expectations of the ways they are most likely to be able to help the patients. It will also avoid doctors using fashionable new treatments which have no proven effect, preventing a repeat of the excessive use in the 19th century of untested physical treatments. In the modern setting such treatments are often referred to as "alternative medicine".

I think that there is a need to train all staff who are working in the community to a level at which they are able to work more independently than they did in the institution. Visiting people in their homes for most of the time and coming back to perhaps to a resource centre for team meetings, means that staff have got to be able to take decisions on their own; that goes for psychiatric trainees, community psychiatric nurses and all other disciplines engaged in the task of community care.

Now training, of course, does not stop with the qualification or appointment to a consultant post in the case of a psychiatrist. It needs to go on, throughout professional life. The Royal College of Psychiatrists is now rapidly developing a continuing medical education programme (CME) for psychiatrists, some of whom may have trained 20 years ago, and may have practised in mental hospitals ever since. It is essential that these kinds of continuing education programmes go on, not just for doctors but for all professions engaged in mental health care because treatments and systems are changing very rapidly.

It is important to keep CME (or continuing professional development - CPD) local and accessible to fully qualified practitioners by means of case conferences and Journal clubs and this means keeping the training relevant to the practice in the community. Peer group support is also crucial and I think resource centres can play an important part in this respect. Professionals working relatively independently, in patients homes for much of the time, need to be coming back to check their practice against that of their peers regularly, and they need to feel that they have a support system in a way that was informally available in the old institutions where staff met more often.

Training in the use of Mental Health Act is very important. There has been some criticism of the Royal College of Psychiatrists about what's perceived as the inadequacy of training in the Mental Health Act. That criticism has come about largely because we only examine on the *principles* of mental health law in our membership examination, which is because different countries within the U.K. have different Mental Health Acts. However, all the time that psychiatrists are in training they are being trained in the apprenticeship system by several consultants consecutively, and as part of that they are being trained in the procedures of the Act of the country in which they're training. We do not therefore believe there to be serious problems in psychiatrist use of the Act.

I want to point out some other difficulties in continuing education and post-graduate education in the community, some of which we are having to face at the moment around the country. Many of the mental hospitals have very large and very valuable stocks of books and journals and very well organised library facilities. Its not possible to take a library and divide it between dispersed sites (e.g; take twelve per cent of it and put it in a community mental health resource centre along with twelve per cent of a librarian's time) because libraries don't work like that. In order to continue to understand research, to continue to keep up with the literature and so on libraries have to be organised in such a way that all professions working in the community can have good access to them, and that may mean having a little greater expenditure on information technology to enable staff to get in touch with a centralised library resource at any time of the day and in addition to have a few bench books locally available in community mental health resource centres. How to protect libraries is a crucial unresolved educational issue in dispersed community services.

A couple of words about other professions - general practitioners in particular. The Royal College of General Practitioners has had a very good scheme for many years but only forty per cent of general practitioners have had any active training at post-graduate level in mental health. With the advent of general practice fund holding where GPs are not only providers of primary mental health care but also purchasers of secondary care, there is a pressing need to make sure that more general practitioners have access to good quality training schemes in psychiatry and for more of them to hold Senior House Officer jobs in psychiatry during their training. This would promote a genuine dialogue between the primary care team and the secondary team and GP fund holders would be better informed and thus able to purchase services from the secondary care team which are well validated and have been shown to be effective.

For this reason the Royal College of Psychiatrists, is now actively planning a diploma in community psychiatry, mainly for general practitioners who've done a brief period of training in psychiatry and who want to have some accreditation and be able to test their own knowledge against an examination procedure. It is hoped that this will encourage more general practitioners to do psychiatry as part of their post-graduate training and that it will increase the number of trained professionals on the ground.

Another group of doctors who need more information and more training to fulfil their functions in the reorganised health service, are public health doctors. The vast majority of public health doctors have no post-graduate experience in mental health and yet some of them have a crucial, role in advising the purchasers of services about their priorities in terms of purchasing mental health services. It is therefore extremely important that public health doctors should be better trained in the realities of mental health service provision than perhaps they have been in the past.

PREPARING THE PROFESSIONS FOR COMMUNITY CARE - NURSES

ANNE JARVIE

First let me put what I say in the context of considerable achievement in the past, with exciting examples of flexibility, innovation and development in moving forward nursing practice in the field of mental health in response to changing clients' needs and expectations. Less than 40 years ago in the mid 50s, the first Community Psychiatric Nurse (CPN) began an outreach service from Warlingham Park Mental Hospital in Epsom, Surrey. In the 60s the matron at Crichton Royal Hospital, Dumfries stated publicly that her main task was outside the hospital, breaking down prejudices and trying to change the misconceptions which surrounded mental illness and mental health problems. It is now recognised that CPNs provide a valuable service, a service which is of value to the clients and is valued by general practitioners and consultants alike.

Nurses pioneered industrial therapy and recreational therapy in many hospitals when it was realised that employment and preparation for return to employment and life in the community was crucial to recovery from mental illness. Nurses became involved in token economy schemes and in the inculcation of budgetary and everyday living skills which, as we all know, are vital to survival in the community. I would venture to claim that nurses have, over the last 3 decades, pioneered many developments in psychiatric care and in doing so have demonstrated their ability to adapt and respond to change.

Mental health nurses are now working in a very wide range of specialities and settings; in wards, day hospitals, hostels, prisons, clinics and in the home. And of course with the elderly with dementia, that most severe and distressing mental illness which places stress on the elderly person, the family and the non-professional and professional carers. In other words, psychiatric nurses are to be found in virtually every branch of the service where nursing care is required and quite a few have carved out worthy careers in the social work profession.

Indeed, as I go around Scotland, I have seen excellent examples of collaborative working. In Tayside, nurses seconded into social work departments enabling social workers and nurses to work together in developing assessment tools and care management. They are learning from, and sharing with, each other - a model that should be emulated. In Moray, I was impressed with the attitude and collaboration of social services and health services at both senior and junior level. I could go on.

Nurses have an important part to play in purchasing. It is said that the main functions of purchasing authorities are to have vision, ability to analyse, ability to develop creative specifications, total quality management, financial management and negotiation and the Audit Commission suggested that there are 3 skill areas that require to be developed to fulfil the purchasing function: data collection of local needs; identification of services to meet the needs; and contracting skills. There is no doubt that nurses, by their practical knowledge gained from working directly with patients and local communities, combined with their management skills, are in a good position to make a valuable contribution in the assessment of health needs and the commissioning of services. Currently, we have nurses in all purchasing teams who, with other members of the team, are coming to grips with the purchasing task and developing the necessary skills.

What I am interested to see develop is the involvement of nurses, midwives and health visitors in the process, especially in the areas of needs assessment and the decisions about the appropriate patterns of service to meet those needs, which of course includes involvement in joint planning with local authorities. It is my view that it is possible to achieve this by secondments. The secondment of a psychiatric nurse to purchasing teams would ensure knowledgeable and practical input to the vision for the mental health service, the analysis of the data and the development of a creative specification which would include realistic and achievable quality components. This would also allow the secondees the opportunity to view mental health and community care from an area-wide perspective and from the purchaser's viewpoint and would contribute to their own personal development. They would gain exposure to the issues surrounding making community care happen via purchasing and joint working, and this would be invaluable to them, no matter what career aspirations they had as individuals.

At the provider end, it is essential that we have highly skilled directors of nursing who are comfortable round the Trust board table and able to contribute with vision on the "how" to make community care happen. The director of nursing must be a real leader who values staff, communicates well, recognises the importance of continuing education and above all is a risk taker who promotes the development of nursing practice. Communication skills are vital because, as we all know, this is the key to managing change. I am happy to say that the Management Development Group are working with me on developing programmes to assist the Executive Director of Nursing to fulfil her role.

But above all in the mental health field, it is essential that the Director of Nursing and her social work colleagues work closely together to develop a shared vision and, if possible, agree a common set of values that cross boundaries of health and social care and facilitate patient-centred care. They should devote time and effort to understand the role of each profession - where there is overlap, and where the key differences lie, and develop implementation programmes which ensure that continuity of care is achieved and that overlaps and gaps become a thing of the past. They should negotiate with each other on the issue of making the best use of available skills. In particular, they should promote the community care agenda and what it means for both professions, together.

Nurses and doctors have traditionally worked closely together, yet we still do not always understand the contribution each can make. It is important that the dialogue is continued and each can make reassessed. Shared care is vital if gaps are to be avoided.

And the Director of Nursing Services requires to concentrate on the maintenance of high quality service for those who require institutional care, while ensuring that adequate resources are available to support those patients who transfer to community settings and require continued support and care from healthcare workers. She needs to consider carefully what new skills are required and discuss with education colleagues any required re-orientation and/or re-training required for the new style service. I believe that psychiatric nurses are likely to have most of the necessary practical and technical skills and that it is change in attitude that requires to be addressed.

Much work has been done already to address the education and training needs of psychiatric nurses to ensure safe and high quality practice in a variety of settings, but programmes will require to be kept under review to ensure that they remain appropriate in a changing world. In its proposals to the government for new preparation for practice, Project 2000, the United Kingdom Central Council was particularly aware of the need to prepare nurses and midwives to provide care in the community and of the World Health Organisation's proposals for Health for All by the Year 2000.

Nurses who have undertaken Project 2000 courses in the mental health branch will be well prepared to provide mental care in the community at staff nurse level. However, the success to taking forward the new style NHS and community care relies on good understanding and collaborative and trusting teamwork. Most nurses are prepared in colleges of nursing and midwifery and so do not have the opportunity to share learning, student life and experience, with the other health professional students and with social work students. This must change in my view.

Nurses who have been practising in a hospital setting for many years may need assistance to practice in a community setting. Mental health nurses are a versatile group who already have the necessary professional skills and for them the period of adaptation and preparation required to be able to practice in the community may not be extensive but each hospital nurse will bring different experiences to the community and so I believe adaptation programmes require to be tailored on an individual basis. Scottish Vocational Qualifications (SVQs) in care can equip care assistants to work in hospital and community settings. Consideration should be given by medical, social and nursing colleagues as to the appropriate duties and responsibilities of care assistants.

What is very clear is that when transferring patients into the community, purchasers and providers will need to identify the new skills hospital staff will have to acquire in order to support patients now being cared for in the community and ensure that contracts make provision for any training and re-training required.

The greatest need is re-orientation with new kinds of teams - teams that are much more multi-disciplinary, which include the person being cared for, their non-professional carers, as well as social workers, doctors, nurses, pharmacists and representatives from housing departments and others. This allows the focus to be on the individual patient and client, the assessed needs and examination of skills required to meet those needs and who within the team has those skills or who can most easily acquire them; it may be appropriate for the family or for the patient or client themselves to have their skills extended. There is a need for the team to learn together and to acknowledge that the client may well be the greatest source of information, and knowledge about themselves.

There is the need for openness, trust and respect within the team and a willingness to explore the boundaries of each professional together. The "Scope of Professional Practice" for nurses issued by the United Kingdom Central Council is, to quote Colin Ralph, "a liberating document". It is up to nurses to take up the challenge and examine the boundaries of their practice and in partnership those of the other professionals, and work together to ensure that the right skills are available to individual patients and clients while achieving this with as few contacts as possible, but that must not be at the expense of having the necessary expertise available. This is the thinking behind the Named Nurse Charter commitment - that is, by naming an individual to be responsible for assessing, planning and evaluating care, meaningful relationships are established between client and professional, communications are improved and continuity of care and carer is achieved.

And finally, have we nearly got to the stage where the balance of power has shifted from the professionals to their clients and patients?

A PERSPECTIVE ON COMMUNITY CARE - THE KENT EXPERIENCE

MR. PETER GILROY

It is important to recognise that we have moved a long way during the last 30 years but there is still a long way to go particularly with regard to professional and public attitudes towards people who suffer from mental ill health.

Mental illness by its nature is profoundly disempowering and the caring professions can sometimes be inward-looking, more concerned about status, hierarchy, professional careers and inter-professional squabbles about boundaries.

At worst this compounds the sense of helplessness which for some has convinced them that they are victims of professional services, their circumstances made worse rather than better through professional intervention. The consequences for many in recent years has been anger and disenchantment with both the system and professional attitudes.

Being somewhat more specific for a moment, when a decision has been made to close an institution, staff fears about their career, their status, their conditions, "Will I have a job?" "Can I cope with this change?" are extremely important questions and need expression and a clear managerial strategy. Nevertheless, by the same token, one has to recognise the user and family's perspective. Obviously if one does not provide a caring environment to staff, it is unlikely that they will have the ability to provide sufficient attention and care for patients/users and their families. Getting the balance right is difficult at the best of times.

I can remember the development of a particular community mental health centre which highlighted how professional power and perception can get in the way of core objectives.

The Community Mental Health Centre (according to users) had been designed by professionals for professionals - doctors, nurses, social workers and psychologists - who were more concerned about the size of their offices, the furniture and equipment, etc. and their own status than about the concerns expressed by patients/users. Users were obviously worried about access, flexibility, the facility of having three meals per day, bathing, laundry and other practical based services within the community. The outcome of this crisis was a total redesign of the Mental Health Centre which fundamentally reduced offices and increased the facilities available to users. The process was not without pain and fundamental questioning of professional attitudes.

Getting priorities right is not an easy task, but it is one of the overriding issues because it has a profound effect on the use of resources and their effectiveness; half-an-hour in a well-heeled office sited within a community mental health centre once a month is not the critical success factor that sustains people with long-term mental ill-health or manages risk on behalf of the general public.

More important is whether there is long-term practical support, warmth, food, a place to live, continuity and sensible professional support systems. The care management approach provides an effective means of ensuring both proper accountability and continuity of care for those people who are a serious risk to themselves or others. Public credibility in our ability to manage risks is the challenge of the 1990s.

Our professional wants sometimes distort overall priorities with regard to resource distribution and therapeutic interventions so that we do not achieve or demonstrate the favourable outcomes required to support people with the greatest needs within the community.

The service at times moves without any sense of direction and professional time is spent on fashionable therapeutic themes - usually with the 'unhappy well' in a wonderful ivory tower type culture - whilst the core objectives, ie ensuring time, effort and skilled resources are addressing the needs of people and their families with long term mental ill-health, are left unaddressed. Therapeutic interventions should be clearly understood both by users and the professional organisations involved in their delivery, they must be accessible and outcome-driven.

Managers and practitioners need on occasions to stand back and view their service from a user perspective. If we continue to drive and develop community provision from an entirely professional view, the balance and style of service will inevitably favour professional needs, not those of users or their families.

The Government's key objectives with regard to community care are summarised in Table 1. It can be seen that there was an expectation that carers' needs would be met and that the best use of resources would be made through a mixed economy of care with the aim of seeking the best possible outcomes for users.

Application of these objectives within Kent

Kent is one of the largest Social Services Departments in England. Its budget in 1994 will be in excess of £224 million. Its population is 1.6 million people, with rising numbers of the under 8s and significant increases over the next six years [40 per cent plus] of the over 80s. Kent is a mixture of outer London conurbations and rural and coastal townships; it is also a major European gateway which has further social implications. The social services department has a very high public profile with over 50,000 contacts a day.

Forty four per cent of direct service expenditure (Figure 1) is purchased from the independent social care sector. It is important to note that this part of the budget is cash and not tied to staff or buildings. The independent social care sector in Kent is large; (Figure 2)it cares for over 23,000 people within Kent. There are over 1,000 residential facilities, 44 domiciliary (home care) contractors, and 12 assessment contractors. This is the 4th year of substantial purchasing and the department has gone through a major cultural shift (Figure 3).

The structure of the service involves a purchaser/provider split, but it is not 'pure' because the purchasers still have partial providing functions. The main purchasing of the Department is concentrated at the point of delivery through our practitioners, care managers and social workers. We have a dedicated stand-alone business units, called the Occupational Therapy (OT) Bureau, which specialises in community assessment and delivery of OT services. The care managers have to have at least a core professional qualification currently in social work occupational therapy, nursing or physiotherapy. This is complemented by modular training which has been developed within the colleges in Kent; We have set up a consortia of both public and private sector agencies - 'Kent Qualified'- which is an accredited centre for NVQ (National Vocational Qualification) assessment and verification.

Kent Social Services works closely with health colleagues across all services. The health service is also undergoing a great deal of change; there has been a move from six health districts to two health authorities which are mainly concerned with commissioning and purchasing, and a number of provider trusts. There is one FHSA and there is a major development of GP fundholding, which has presented opportunities and challenges in the way that we plan for services and work together.

How does all this work in Kent? Our first overriding objective in providing services is that they be provided quickly and flexibly, tailored around an individual or their family's needs, offering choice and maximising innovation where appropriate and purchasing services within the mixed economy of care. In an attempt to meet this objective, major investment in information technology has been required; £14 million of capital investment and a revenue commitment of over £3 million per year.

An adequate information infrastructure is required if there is to be a shift from the 'take it or leave it' approach, (fixing people into existing systems of care): to a needs-led approach (purchasing to meet the needs of individuals and families): manual systems will not suffice. Consequences of this change in approach are:-

*   greater choice

*   an inevitable competition with the independent and in-house suppliers of services.

*   a shift of power between the user/carers and professionals involved which requires a sophisticated system to manage the process.

Currently every practitioner has his/her own terminal with access to data on community resources as well as on caseloads and budgets, with the power to allocate and purchase resources from a range of providers. This has provided a powerful framework which has facilitated a needs-led approach to service delivery.

It has also meant, probably for the first time, practitioners and users having up-to-date information about both informal and formal resources across the locality, district and county. By March 1994 care managers will have access to formal residential and nursing home data (by postal code) for the whole of the UK.

Community resource information is of critical importance in community care services. It empowers users, it provides choice, and offers professionals comparative costs and values. It also brings a degree of clarity regarding the outcomes expected of any particular service. Information about services is of critical importance in making community care work. This information needs to be readily available to service users, not just to professionals.

In order to do this we commissioned an independent agency to provide software packages (updated monthly) on all community resources, formal and informal, public, voluntary, private and health. This database is now up and running and on care managers' terminals. It will be available to general practitioners, district nurses and health visitors as well as other specialists. (Target: Summer 1994).

As a consequence of devolving cash limits and a high degree of delegation we have had to create eligibility criteria for services, identify priorities and make public statements about what we can provide and what we cannot. Targeting of resources has been the inevitable consequence. Users and practitioners have had a profound influence on the shape and style of services and have responded constructively to a more open approach about the opportunities cash purchasing has brought, and its limitations.

At the present time we have 1,000 purchasers within the Department which is providing diversity and a richness in innovation. This would not have been possible if the Department had not pursued a devolved system of both delegation and resource distribution.

In spite of the benefits there have been criticisms that the Department is organising and running services based on commercial principles. It is true that we work within a business planning framework, identifying activity levels against costs with clear outcomes and performance indicators which reflect the objectives identified within the community care plans. It is also true that everyone within the organisation is on performance related pay. However, we have not lost our value base and believe that we would stand up against any public agency in the country, both in terms of standards, values and quality.

Given the level of devolvement of resources and power to practitioners, is it now difficult to keep any strategic context in place? The social services department is divided into five strategic and operational subsidiary areas. In each one there are commissioners who control the purchasing, through practitioners, of services for adults and children. It is here where the convergence of service and strategic issues takes place ie. community care planning, joint commissioning, joint agency work, aggregation of user needs etc.

Demographic analysis and management control data assist in identifying strategic priorities as do the central and local government policy directives. The process within each area is also fed directly from users and practitioners, particularly the identification of gaps in provision against prevailing needs.

If a practitioner decides with a family that there is a deficit in service, for example where the family still feels that certain types of service would have met their needs more appropriately, this deficit would be entered into the local computer terminal. This information is then aggregated on a six monthly basis and is part of the information jigsaw that informs planning and service development. The system is not perfect but it is becoming more and more sophisticated and it is certainly having a profound effect on the shape and type of service currently being delivered.

There is clearly a closer partnership with families with this approach. The capability of individualised purchasing as opposed to block contracting makes a statement about putting family and individual needs first. We are giving the public/users some control over and choice about the type, style and quality of services received.

This year, 1993/94, flexibility has been the hallmark. 146,000 assessments and 30,000 care packages have highlighted a major shift, particularly regarding support at home schemes, respite services and a range of individual variations developed with the voluntary and private sector. (£100 million will be spent on services provided by the independent sector in 1994). Diversification by providers has been very significant indeed. I believe it is because individual practitioners have been able to negotiate directly changes in services in response to clients' needs.

To recap, my underlying theme:

1. A needs-led approach to mental health services means an absolute requirement of proper support systems for practitioners and the organisation. This requires long-term strategic investment, preferably on a multi-agency basis.

2. It does mean a change of emphasis and new ways of working in practice, with greater clarity on objectives, priorities and accountabilities. It is particularly important to ensure continuity of care.

3. Information is power, and information about resources is critical to success in any community care service, with access for both users and carers as well as professionals.

4. Greater understanding of costs and values brings benefits to the organisation's use of resources. Competition inevitably brings about change in the providers of services and a cultural shift for the professions involved. This, however, is a subtle process and happens through negotiation, not a macho approach to contracting.

5. Major flexibility in managing service change to meet needs is one of the outcomes of devolved management. Managers of services have to be more concerned about outcome rather than process.

6. Multi-disciplinary training is of greater importance than ever before, as is the need to understand the implications for social services, health service and community housing in all its forms, particularly the shifting position with local authorities and the increasing role of housing associations.

7. The shift to community care services is not a cheap option. An existing case makes the point: (Table 1).The lady has a community care package which involves more than one agency. She is highly dependent and has been diagnosed as suffering from dementia. The cost per week now exceeds £270.00 (this does not include medical and nursing costs). This is higher than the cost of an average residential place. As community care packages become more complex the costs will inevitably rise and this could be the significant pressure in the next five years for all services, but particularly on specialist services like mental health. Rising costs, and governments of the day and the general public expecting more and more for less will force managers, politicians and the professions into greater clarity about effectiveness, eligibility and priorities.

Experience in community mental health centres in this country and the USA shows an increasing tendency to disenfranchise the chronically ill in favour of those conditions which are 'susceptible to change'. This means that many get very little practical help.

A community nurse or social worker popping in once a month to a bed-sit for a cup of tea, or trying to fix individuals into a local day centre for an afternoon a week is not community care and will not be successful. There is a public credibility issue here. Real community care is about taking a long-term interest; being accountable, having the ability to network, access and purchase different kinds of appropriate care; taking a realistic view; and ensuring a sense of continuity both with the family and local primary health services.

A mental health service at its best is holistic by nature and does not isolate itself from all the natural resources existing within any community, (employment, housing, income, social support networks). It is my view that care management clearly provides the ability to individualise the assessment process and directly influence resource distribution. It also facilitates imagination, flair and user involvement.

It concerns me that from an organisational point of view that there are now constant pressures to find efficiency savings without an agreement to reinvest these savings in the current service. Nationally we have closed a number of hospitals but it is clear that money has not followed the patient, with flows of revenue disappearing into the black hole of acute services. Policy makers cannot expect managers or specialists in community provision to show innovation with efficient use of resources if revenue is continually plundered year on year.

We are seeing the results of this, sadly, in some of our inner cities. Efficiency savings are fine. However, if they are not coupled with the ability to recycle these savings, they lose purpose and are then seen as cutting services rather than making them more efficient.

Mental health services in the 1990s require vision, determination and a sense of optimism. The best and most effective services are those where a partnership exists between practitioners, users and managers and where there is a clear understanding and expectation from providers across agencies of working together to provide the best possible services within the resources available to them.

Table 1

CARE MANAGEMENT

COSTING ANALYSIS - 11.04.93 - 18.04.93

Consumer - MISS MAUD SCOTT

SERVICE	UNIT COST £	NO. UNITS	TOTAL COST £
Care Worker (Day)	8.00	14	112.00
Care Worker (Eves)	13.00	7	91.00
Meals on Wheels	1.60	14	22.40
Home Help (Domestic)	3.50	2	7.00
Voluntary Driver	9.90	1	9.90
Day Centre	23.50	1	23.50
Community Alarm System	5.00	1	5.00

SERVICE TOTAL   **£270.80**
(excludes Care Management Costs)

Figure 1

Kent County Council Social Services Department Gross BudgetDistribution 1994-95

Total Gross Budget £225.7m

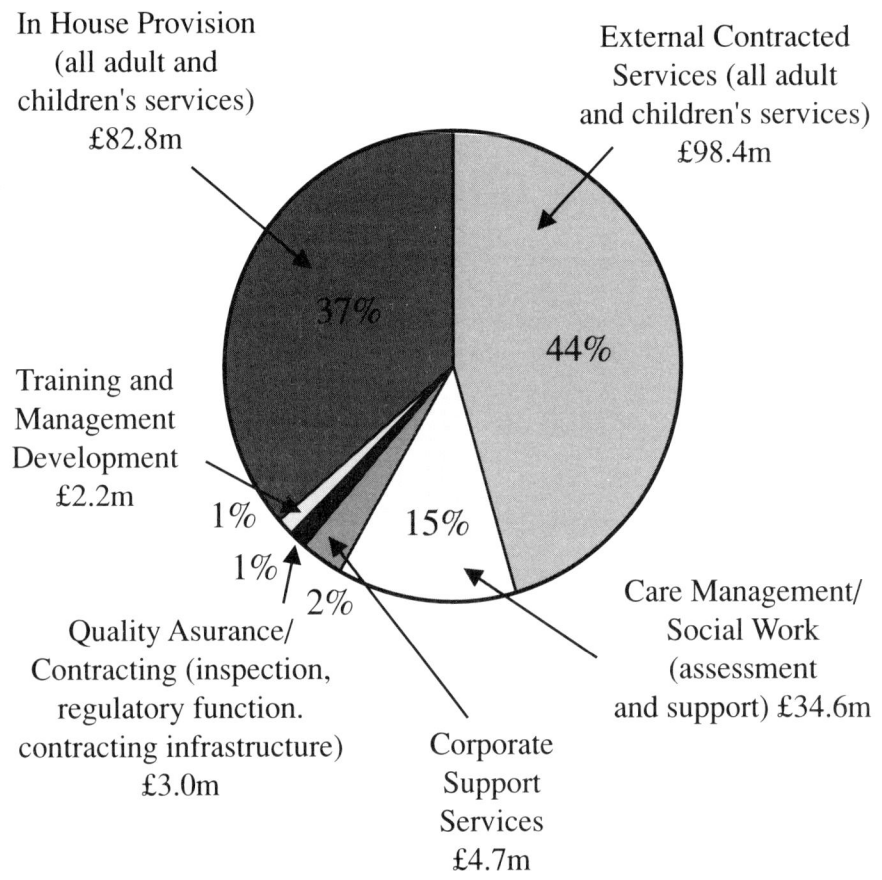

In House Provision (all adult and children's services) £82.8m

External Contracted Services (all adult and children's services) £98.4m

Training and Management Development £2.2m

37%

44%

1%

1%

2%

15%

Quality Asurance/ Contracting (inspection, regulatory function. contracting infrastructure) £3.0m

Corporate Support Services £4.7m

Care Management/ Social Work (assessment and support) £34.6m

Figure 2

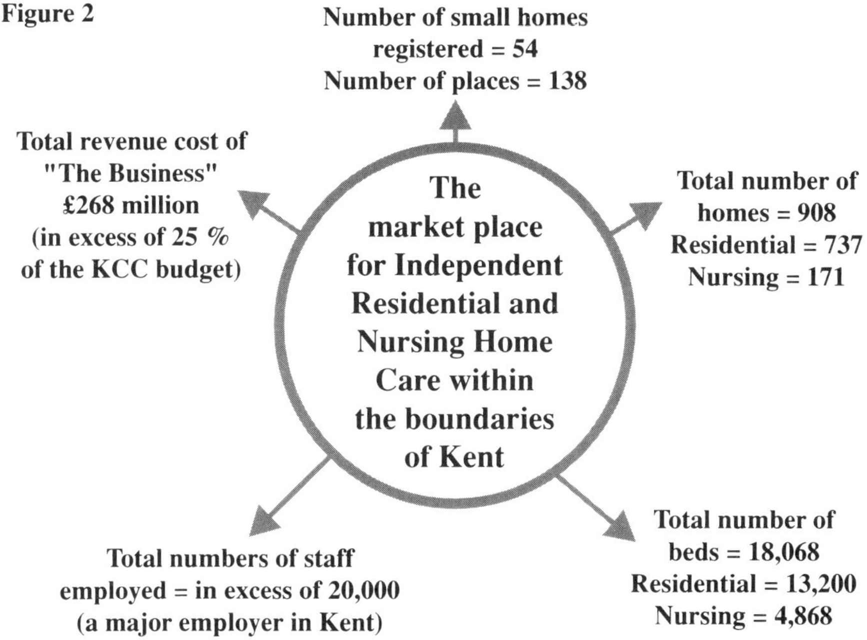

Number of small homes
registered = 54
Number of places = 138

Total revenue cost of
"The Business"
£268 million
(in excess of 25 %
of the KCC budget)

The
market place
for Independent
Residential and
Nursing Home
Care within
the boundaries
of Kent

Total number of
homes = 908
Residential = 737
Nursing = 171

Total number of
beds = 18,068
Residential = 13,200
Nursing = 4,868

Total numbers of staff
employed = in excess of 20,000
(a major employer in Kent)

Figure 3

Kent County Council
Social Services Department

- Strategic/negotiation
- Aggregation of Community needs
- Working within the mixed econonmy of care

**Direct
Service
Provision
Group**

COMMISSIONERS ⟶ CONTRACTING AND
DEVELOPMENT ARM

PURCHASING

CARE MANGERS/SOCIAL WORKERS/OTs

Individualised purchasing
arrangements following
personal assessment

Customer
£100m
(External market)

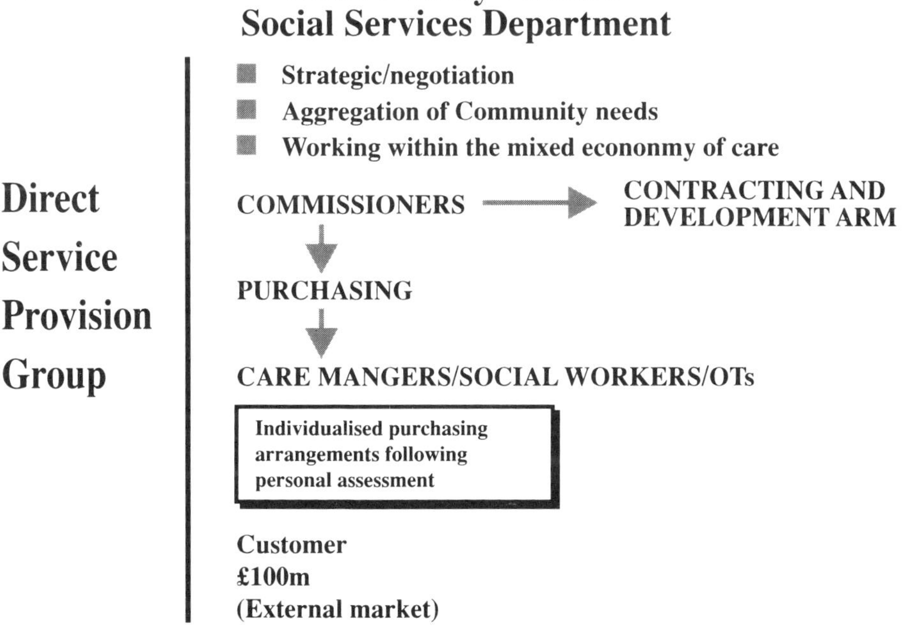

THE CHALLENGES FOR VOLUNTARY ORGANISATIONS

PETER MILLAR

Thank you for giving me the opportunity of addressing you today. Whilst I have liaised with other mental health voluntary organisations in the Glasgow area who are service providers, such as LINK/GAMH, SAMH and the Archdiocese of Glasgow, in respect of this presentation, the comments are ultimately my own although the issues raised are of general interest.

The mental health voluntary organisations face challenges in implementing community care services - advocacy, staff training, the competitive environment inherent in the contracts culture, funding, users' participation and monitoring and evaluation. These issues are important if the best possible service is to be provided in respect of users within a proper funding framework.

For most of this century mental health services have comprised only large remote psychiatric institutions with vested interests maintaining the status quo. Recently there has been an explosion of activity triggered by Griffiths and culminating in the *Caring for People* White Paper and subsequent legislation and guidance. The response to this explosion has varied from area to area in Scotland. In some places there appears to have been little change whilst in others people have been galvanised into positive action.

This latter response has clearly been evident in Greater Glasgow, where over the past few years literally hundreds of long-stay psychiatric hospital residents have been helped to move into new registered residential and day-care schemes in the community managed by voluntary organisations. This is a tribute particularly to the Community Mental Health Unit and the Health Board supported by Social Work and Housing. The recently published *Mental Health Strategy Document* must also be warmly applauded as long as it is properly resourced resulting in a needs-led rather than a service-led reality, put into place with the proper timing.

In another chapter the Greater Glasgow Mental Health Unit confirm that the Mental Health Strategy proposes that comprehensive community mental health services would be in place prior to the closure of Gartloch and Woodilee Hospitals. That is clearly excellent and very reassuring, but is there a danger that once those institutions have been closed, that these community mental health services may be gradually eroded? They would be relatively soft targets for future contraction. **It is important therefore, that**

funding for these community care services be ring-fenced on a long term basis to properly support the long-term needs of users and carers.

The voluntary sector has a lot of experience in community care for people with mental illness and their families and has historically been very innovative in providing community care services. The health sector in contrast has historically mainly invested in maintaining people in remote Victorian institutions, keeping people whom society viewed "out of their minds" - out of sight.

The local authority social work department occasionally dealt in the past with individuals with mental illness during an acute psychotic episode. This was usually when a mental health officer was involved in the person's detention in hospital; the reason for this being that no other adequately supported alternative was made available. Nevertheless a focused service had at least been provided to deal with an acute and highly visible need. However, historically, people with long term mental illness have not had their needs met largely because their "mental illness" was not properly acknowledged; their problems instead being categorised as probation, child care, matrimonial proceeding cases etc. This was a result of generic social work which has had difficulty in focusing upon each client group.

The above situation is now changing, for instance where de-institutionalisation from long-stay hospital is taking place, health and social work (with housing)3 authorities are reshaping their services and targeting energies and resources. These resources include new forms of funding such as bridging finance and mental illness specific grant aimed at providing better community care services for people with mental illness and their carers. But this focused approach is relatively new.

Many voluntary sector organisations have had a focused approach towards community care services for people with mental illness and their carers for many decades. Some organisations have taken a campaigning role whereas others have elected to be primarily service-providers.

Until relatively recently voluntary organisations have had plenty of time for lateral thinking on how to be most creative and innovative in setting-up services. In the current situation rapid expansion of the voluntary sector could increasingly impose pressure to replicate proven "models" without enough fresh innovative thinking. As many voluntary organisations are growing significantly in size, there is a real risk of them becoming bureaucratic and remote from users; of insidiously meeting the needs of "the staff" to the detriment of users needs. Areas such as user participation, advocacy, training and monitoring and evaluation are crucially important in ensuring that that does not happen.

There is a growing trend for voluntary organisations to be more like businesses than they were before and this is entirely appropriate; care management and resource management are inextricably linked. However, organisations must remain fundamentally user-centred if they are to fulfil their role. The freshness, flexibility, spontaneity and challenging approach which typifies the voluntary sector should be retained if the needs of users are to be met.

The role of the voluntary sector as an advocate for users and carers is arguably also in jeopardy because of a potential conflict of interest in situations where the voluntary organisation is funded by the public sector. This issue is not, however, unique to the voluntary sector. It nevertheless remains a challenge in ensuring that the rights and needs of users continue to be of paramount importance.

The purchaser provider split is offering new challenges to the voluntary sector in taking up opportunities for collaborative working, with Regional Council Social Work Departments, Health Boards, NHS Trusts - and other voluntary organisations. We have much to learn from each other and owe it to users and carers to work closely together towards providing comprehensive, pertinent and complementary services.

In Glasgow several of the mental health service providers have recently established the "Glasgow Voluntary Organisations Service Providers Consortium" and the Richmond Fellowship Scotland is involved also in similar groups in Grampian and Ayrshire.

Staff training is extremely important as it has a direct relationship with quality of care provision. As voluntary organisations increasingly recruit health care staff to work in community care settings, training plays a vitally important re-orientation role.

The Richmond Fellowship Scotland has established 6 supported accommodation with day-care schemes in the past 18 months (see Tables 1 & 2). The vast majority of staff in these schemes have come from a health care background - usually hospital-based psychiatric nurses. These individuals have been recruited because of their personalities, motivation, life experience and work experience and training. They have great potential as care and development staff. **However,** there is considerable training required to re-orientate these previous hospital based health care workers towards a community-based social care approach. We are finding this a most satisfying exercise but it takes time, energy and the necessary funding to make it work properly.

The contracts culture imposes a competitive environment. This can be healthy as it can be argued that it encourages efficiency and a striving to provide better quality services; it also introduces alternative styles, and choices, and provides a mixed market where different providers can learn from each other. However, there is a risk in any competitive tendering environment that quality **could** be reduced by voluntary organisations:

(i)   **inappropriately** cutting costs of a Scheme to win a tender or by;

(ii)   **inappropriately** proposing increased numbers of clients/residents to be served and securing unit cost advantages via economies of scale - thus reducing overall scheme costs, but also, for instance, destroying the homeliness which can be achieved by a small Residential Care Scheme. The contracts culture could also set voluntary organisations against each other. An important challenge for these organisations will be learning to live with competition (which is not new, but is heightened in a competitive tendering environment) and also seek ways to complement and learn from each other. As indicated above, voluntary organisations are taking steps towards doing this in several areas in Scotland.

Funding: has been a perennial problem for voluntary organisations with the insecurity of funding being provided on a year-to-year basis. A real advantage of the contracts culture is that multi-year contracts provide greater stability and opportunities to plan ahead.

There is a challenge for us all in establishing community-care services. Its name is **Prejudice.** This is apparent in the Not In My Back Yard (NIMBY) Syndrome.

We **all** have a collective responsibility in dealing with this matter, such as:

(i)   providing more "good news" promoting mental health and publishing successful community care initiatives;

(ii)   the Scottish Office closely examining the **planning legislation and guidance** which is available to planning authorities to determine whether further action is required to ensure that these are sufficiently clear and cannot be used as vehicles for obstructing people with disabilities from living in the community;

(iii)   increasing efforts to help integrate people with mental illness into a variety of services enjoyed by the mainstream public which should provide an educational experience due to direct contact being enabled.

Although the final area to mention concerns **monitoring and evaluation** it would be wrong to regard these activities as low priority luxuries.

Funding agencies, "contract compliance monitors" and the social work departments' registration and inspection staff fulfil valued functions. There may be advantage in enhancing that external evaluation by establishing a "peer group" audit arrangement with another voluntary organisation in the field.

Historically service users have tended to be passive receivers of care, particularly in the power-hierarchy of the psychiatric hospitals, but this could also happen in a community based social care facility. Size and setting are factors but the key determinant is **attitudinal approach** expressed in practice.

*   We need to maintain a strong does of humility. We **don't** know better than users, we just have a **different** view of the world.

*   We must always look, not just at care needs, but also at the development needs, the potentials **of** and the possibilities **for,** the individual user with whom we work.

*   In a spirit of partnership with users we have to find ways of sharing power and control where it really matters. Practical examples of this in my own organisation are:

(i)   in **service planning:** via our users participation group deciding on whether we should develop particular services. We are currently deciding whether to tender for a supported accommodation and day care scheme. If we do proceed, we would invite users to work together with staff in formulating the tender with respect to the proposed operational design of the scheme.

(ii)   in **service delivery:** each time we have a staff vacancy in an existing scheme, users of that scheme are invited to be involved in the preliminary screening of job applicants by meeting with them, and the users then nominate a representative to sit on the interview panel with staff. The logic for this is that users have a vested interest in ensuring we jointly reach the right decision and the corollary is that they share the responsibility if we get it wrong!

In conclusion, I would suggest to you that the not-for-profit making voluntary sector, despite some growing pains, is coming of age. We are keen to work closely with the statutory sector in developing services and I reckon that to a large extent we share the same values of treating people with respect and dignity - and doing our utmost to give them the best possible services the available money can buy.

The voluntary sector has always had a compassionate approach and it is to be hoped that this will be maintained but it has to become hard-headed. This balanced combination of attributes will, be increasingly important as voluntary sector organisations continue to grow in both size and stature.

TABLE 1

STAFFING CHARACTERISTICS:
PROFESSIONALLY QUALIFIED IN SOCIAL WORK/HEALTH CARE

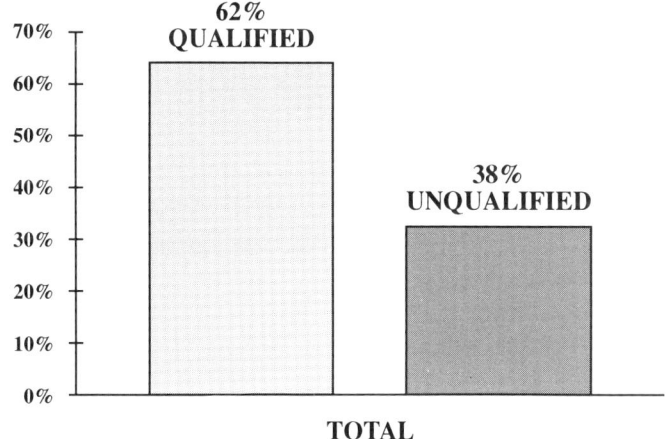

TABLE 2

THE RICHMOND FELLOWSHIP SCOTLAND
SCHEMES STAFFING CHARACTERISITCS:
PROFESSIONAL QUALIFICATIONS/PREVIOUS EMPLOYMENT

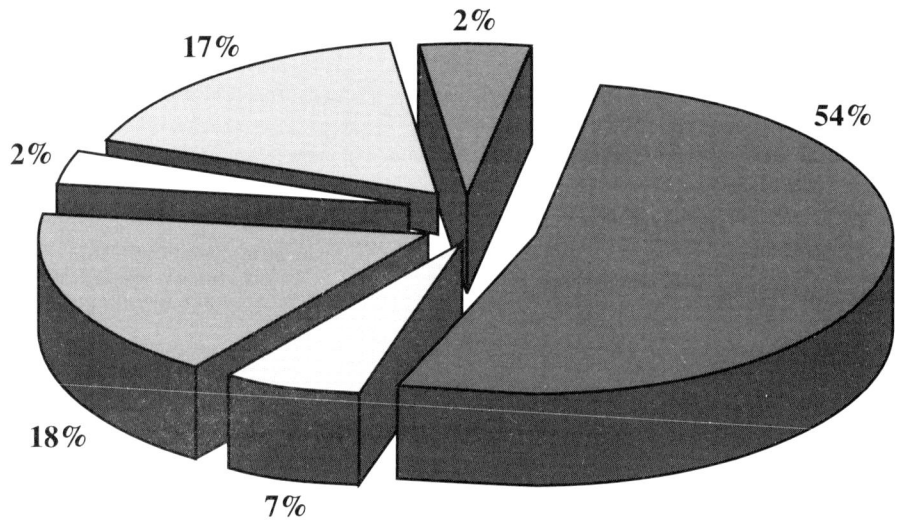

CQSW/CSS (Social Work Quals.)   Registered Mental Nurse

Enrolled Nurse   Health Care Asst.

O.T. Asst.   Other

THE CHALLENGES FOR VOLUNTARY ORGANISATIONS

MR. MARTIN SIME

There are many hundreds of voluntary bodies involved in mental health in Scotland, from big national care providers to small, local self help groups. They all have different perspectives on needs and priorities, and they all work in different ways. Diversity is the strength of the voluntary organisations; but it also makes life difficult for planners and purchasers since the voluntary sector is not rationally organised. Voluntary organisations rarely speak with one voice, but I will attempt to bring together a collection of issues and concerns which represent as near as possible to a voluntary sector agenda.

Voluntary organisations have major criticisms of the statutory sector; that the speed of change is too slow; that the voluntary sector are offered inadequate resources to run vital services; that the sectors contributions are not rated seriously and that there's been an absence of strategic vision from the centre.

There are also criticisms of the voluntary sector. A recent Home Office publication, the Centris Report, painted a gloomy picture of the voluntary sector as over-bureaucratic, overpaid and increasingly out of touch. It called for the abolition of charitable status and the division of the voluntary sector into campaigning groups on the one hand and service providers on the other. Tax relief would be available to the latter, but only on the basis of performance appraisal; the government has rejected these recommendations.

The voluntary sector has been likened with Columbus - not sure about where he was going, not knowing where he is when he gets there and not at all clear about where he's been when he returns. But it didn't matter since the journey has been made with other people's money.

The voluntary sector cannot be pigeonholed in this way. It is not a corporate entity and that is at least in part because government does not want it to be. Our collaborative and co-operative instincts founder on the realities of purchaser/provider relationships and the market place which governments and health boards have created. In the purchaser/provider world competition is expected and monopolies, cartels or consortia are discouraged. The long-standing partnership of the voluntary organisations with local government and our history of sharing and inter-agency agreements has been sorely tested, by the competition for re-provision contracts.

The voluntary sector is, by and large, committed to the mixed economy of care but will never accept the imposition of an enterprise led and profit driven culture. The term, "independent sector", is not acceptable in its rather crude effort to bring the voluntary and private sectors together. The voluntary sector's broader aims include trying to influence what is purchased as well as actually trying to be the provider.

Taking the voluntary sector seriously is a particular challenge to mental health service professionals. The vast majority of community mental health services in Scotland are actually run by voluntary agencies and yet the sector is often seen as peripheral.

In Scotland the role of statutory agencies in community care, especially in residential care is unclear. Are they to be commissioners, enablers, purchasers only or will they - as the Scottish chapter in the White Paper said, continue to be major and direct providers?

So competing with statutory sector empires, when they hold the purse strings, creates particular problems for the voluntary sector. It would help if a non-statutory target were set. Money is well spent in the voluntary sector. There is no private profit; the sector has a wealth of experience and ideas; people tend to be committed, both individually and collectively through their organisations; the organisations are known for being able to act quickly and to harness energies and skills from health, social work and beyond; and the voluntary sector can often bring in additional resources - governmental, european, housing and private donations - to the table. In view of the size of the task in Scotland of implementing the changes, there is a need to change attitudes towards the voluntary sector and for investment in its capacity to be the leading provider in the future.

Joint planning has not proved to be satisfactory as far as the voluntary organisations are concerned; planning seems to run parallel to, and unconnected with, actual service development. It's difficult to see why the voluntary sector should devote its scarce resource and energies to planning until we can be assured that tangible results will follow.

We need to acknowledge and analyze what's gone wrong in the past. Why has joint planning and joint finance failed to deliver since 1985? If we knew and recognised the answer, we probably wouldn't make the same mistake again.

There are only 20 or so major providers of community mental health services in the voluntary sector in Scotland. There are several hundreds of other groups, often local, many of them based on self-help or with particular focus, and one of the many challenges which the voluntary sector faces is the need to put aside rivalries and territorialism, which are being stimulated by the market economy, and to build on the basic respect which we have for what we are all doing. I would like to see more collaborative work, involving the big providers and local groups, bringing forward new ideas based on the experience of those closest to the ground, allied to the greater organisational capacity of the major agencies.

The voluntary sector is increasingly concerned about losing its campaigning edge. This challenge takes 2 distinct forms: firstly, the concern that increasing service provision will swamp the public advocacy origins of many groups and secondly, that agencies will become frightened to rock the boat or bite the hand that feeds them.

At another level, the greater involvement of voluntary organisations in actually providing services, the more it seems to me that the balance tips against their legitimacy as advocates for their own service users. We may yet find local authorities taking up the role of advocates against voluntary sector providers!

The biggest challenge facing the sector is to practice what it preaches in relation to user involvement. Some of us undoubtedly do risk becoming funding led and service driven, without devoting the space or energy to making sure that we enable the people we work with to take control. User involvement in voluntary sector services is an absolute necessity for the future health and vitality of voluntary organisations.

The other issue is to do with the scale of new developments. It has taken voluntary organisations nearly 2 decades to develop around a thousand supported accommodation places across Scotland. Whilst we applaud the recent Community Care Implementation Unit targets of 600 transfers a year until the turn of the century, this scale of change is a real challenge for the voluntary sector; the scale of operation of the sector will need to be increased if we are to play a major role in meeting this target.

The dangers for us, are that the decay of bureaucracy will set in - that models will be replicated inappropriately and that innovation and campaigning, which are the hallmarks and tradition of a vibrant and independent voluntary sector, will take a back seat. Our agencies will become awash with administrators, contract negotiators, lawyers and that modern day scourge of creativity and vitality, management accountants. Of course, we do need to acquire skills, expertise and successful methodologies from both the public and private sectors but voluntary organisations must pick and choose judiciously and take care not to absorb too much from any one source, lest the sector loses touch with its original aims and becomes no more than another quango or arm's length agency of government.

To conclude, how will we know, that the vision of a community mental health service is going to become a reality? When the first health board announces that it is spending more in the community than on institutional care; when mental health promotion, mental illness prevention and advocacy receive priority funding; when a group of users make recommendations about service priorities which result in major changes to community care plans; when health boards and social work departments reach a comprehensive agreement about needs, responsibilities, service strategies and funding; and lastly when health and social work invite voluntary agencies into real collective partnerships and pool their resources to address agreed service priorities.

To end on a salutary note, even with the commitment of everyone concerned, it may be more than 6 years from now before many people can benefit from the policy of community care, first announced as John Henderson said yesterday by Enoch Powell in 1959 but reiterated as government policy in an Act of Parliament 3 years ago. Three years or 39 from policy to practice would not be tolerated elsewhere in public and private life and perhaps we might consider whether the targets which have been set, difficult though they might seem at the moment, should themselves be speeded up.

THE CONTRIBUTION OF SERVICE USERS IN THE DESIGN AND IMPLEMENTATION OF SERVICES

MR. PETER CAMPBELL

The idea that service users can be actively involved in making a contribution is a fairly novel idea. Ten years ago there was little involvement of users in the field of mental health 1983 was the year of the Mental Health Act in England and Wales and as far as I am aware service users were not directly involved in any significant way in deciding what went into the Mental Health Act 1983, and that is a major piece of legislation, which concerns everything to do with the provision of mental health services and civil liberties etc. for people in England and Wales. My impression is that the same is true in Scotland of the 1984 Act. That wouldn't be possible today and this is an indication that things have moved on. It is worth remembering that 10 years ago there were actually very few independent user action groups. The voice of the service user was being expressed through the voluntary organisations: organisations in England and Wales like National MIND for example. Sometimes it was being expressed in quite an inadequate way. I remember about this time going down to the National Mind Offices as an isolated individual service user, because I was very concerned about discrimination in employment. I used to go down to the National Mind Office and ask for information about their activities. I expressed the desire to actually do something and have direct access to people who might matter; although I was very courteously treated and given information I was not encouraged. "Well there's nothing really you can do in terms of getting directly involved". Glasgow Link Education and Action on Mental Health Group was the first group of service users I came across which was involved in making a collective contribution to the debate. They made a presentation to the National Mind Conference in 1984. I read about this subsequently down in London, and thought this is the first time I have heard of a Group of users actually getting together and doing something. I wrote to them in Glasgow to find out what was going on. There has been a lot of progress since 1984; voluntary organisations clearly now do represent the concerns of the users much more effectively and there are a large number of independent user action groups, local user action groups around the country. When Survivors Speak Out was founded as a networking organisation in 1986, there were probably about a dozen independent user action groups in the whole of this country. Now there are between 200 and 300 hundred groups. Users around the country are making a wide range of contributions. It is only in the last couple of years, that user action, has actually become credible. Until a couple of years ago, everytime someone like me was on a platform, or speaking in public, we used to preface everything we said, with a five minute explanation of why the audience should be listening to a user in the first place. Now, when there are conferences around the country about user involvement, we seem to spend much less time with the flip charts on the "why involve service users?" topic than we used to and tend to go on to the "How to involve users" question and the problems. Although it is now accepted that there are good reasons for involving service users, the struggle over this issue of credibility continues. Service providers and mental health workers are more happy to think about users as a collection of individuals, who they might be able to empower by giving better information, giving a care programme approach, giving a key worker or giving a care manager than to think of users as a collective, organised movement who are actually getting together and putting forward and lobbying for specific proposals. This is still quite uncomfortable. There is still a feeling that for service users to get organised and form pressure groups, lobbying groups, is not playing the game right. Collective organisations of service users can make a valuable contribution and are doing so already, and this is not simply to do with the design and implementation of services. There are four main areas where users of services are making a contribution. First of all, the planning of services which is being focused on quite a lot as a result of the community care legislation. Secondly, in the area of increasing control over the individual's own care and treatment. There have been some good successes in England, in terms of users being involved in devising their own information packs, self assessment forms, and so on. Thirdly in providing services - this is still a fairly underdeveloped area and fourthly, in changing attitudes. When considering the planning of services, it's important to remember the role of purchasing. Service users can make a contribution directly to purchasers, by being involved in examining the services in their area and making suggestions to purchasers in terms of specifications, by commenting upon contracts and by monitoring services after they are established. There is a good example of this happening in Newcastle, where the Newcastle Mental Health Consumer Group has been funded, and well funded, to give detailed advice to mental health purchasers.

The role of service users in changing attitudes is vitally important and user groups and individuals have already done valuable work in terms of training mental health workers and in addressing public attitudes.

I think one of the most interesting things for me personally, that the user movement has achieved, has been to give people who have experiences of particular problems the chance to get together and talk about their experience and what their lives are about. A good example of this was when the user movement in England and Wales was involved in organising a conference on self injury three years ago. This was the first national conference where people who self-injure had the chance to get up and talk about their experience and also talk to mental health workers who are interested in this field. Since then there has been a similar conference for people with eating distress, people who are diagnosed as having problems like anorexia nervosa or bulimia[1]. There has also been a development called the Hearing Voices network; the group are concerned with redefining what it means to hear voices, how people can actually cope with that experience in a better way, and how to change public perceptions[2].

There are certainly technical difficulties in involving service users; problems about what is the best way of actually involving service users in planning structures, in committees. There are problems about jargon, about language, about the way things are done and about what is the most friendly way of doing things as far as users are concerned. There are problems about the time it takes to organise user contributions. There are questions about resources which are significant. There is also a problem about users and professionals having different agendas. User action groups are concerned with empowering people in their own lives and that may not be very much to do with providing services. People get involved in order to change their own lives, and they may not see much value in sitting on planning committees. They may not want to be involved in interviewing psychiatrists for prospective services. People who provide services, people who work in services, often have well developed agendas and they know what they want service users to do. They have a brief and they want to get service users involved in that brief. Within the user movement, people are developing their own agendas, finding out what they want to do, what they think is important, what they think is good fun to be involved in and there is a danger that because service providers have a stronger agenda, they will actually drag user groups and users into things that users might not actually want to be involved in. Service providers are often concerned about the representation of service users who are members of local groups. Are they actually hearing the voice of the people they want to hear? If service providers want organisations to be representative, then they have got to actually make that clear and they have got to give people the chance to be representative. The user movement has spent a lot of time trying to develop advocacy projects, specifically designed to help people who have difficulty in voicing their concerns, to voice those concerns. It is not because we are not concerned to allow everybody to have a voice, that people currently don't all have a voice.

One other major difficulty is how do you actually ensure that the more radical, the more innovative demands of service users are listening to? In particular, users have some concerns about the length of time it has actually taken for the spontaneous demand for 24 hour crisis services, to actually result in something on the ground. User groups have been asking for this for over 10 years. Asking for services which provide an alternative destination to hospitals, for services which allow them to go through crisis without being medicated out of consciousness. When this is a clear major demand of users of mental health services, why is it taking so long for that to be addressed? There is also a major question about the role of medication in mental health care. It is quite clear from the user movement around the world, that substantial numbers of users want to see services which don't depend totally on medication. There is a divergence between that expression of what users want and what they are actually getting; there is a problem about opening up a discussion about what is the role of medication. For instance do we need to have so many people on such high doses of medication? Do we have to resort to medication in times of crisis? One illustration of the kind of concerns that some of us have is that attempts by the user movement to actually provide support to people who want to withdraw from major tranquillisers is largely an underground operation. There is quite substantial opposition to actually opening up the possibility of services that aren't based on medication and the services are not supporting people who want to withdraw from their medication. If these overall questions aren't actually being addressed, is there really a will to provide a user led service?

REFERENCES

1. Pembroke Louise (editor). Eating Distress: Perspectives from personal experience. Survivors Speak Out, 34 Osnaburgh Street, London NW1 3ND.

2. Hearing Voices Network. c/o MACC, Swan Buildings, 20 Swan Street, Ancoats, Manchester M4 5JW.

THE CONTRIBUTION OF SERVICE USERS IN THE DESIGN AND IMPLEMENTATION OF SERVICES

MR. JIM READ

The key issue in the involvement of service users in the design and implementation of services this: do purchasers and providers really want to hear what service users have to say and are they willing to act to put our good ideas into practice?

In the last few years, there has been a growth of advocacy projects, patients' councils, local user forums and national networks of people who are recipients of psychiatric services. There have been surveys and research projects to find out users' views, and videos produced by people who - to use one memorable self-definition - have experienced services from the wrong side of the drugs trolley.

With all this activity, which has never occurred before on anything like the same scale, a picture is beginning to emerge of what service users want from mental health services. Those involved in self advocacy have very different views from each other about basic issues, such as, is there such a thing as mental illness, is there a role for medication, can compulsory detention in psychiatric hospitals ever be justified? But, despite these fundamental differences of opinion it seems comparatively easy for us to agree the principals on which a mental health service should be based. Firstly, I am going to examine the issues that have been identified under a number of headings - information, choice, accessibility, advocacy, equal opportunities, income and employment, self help and self organisation. This will allow purchasers and providers to consider whether they are prepared to provide a service that service users say they want.

Starting with information: more than anything else, service users want to know about the effects of medication. One extensive survey found that 68% of people who have been prescribed major tranquillisers were not informed about the expected effects.[1] Having been told about these effects, most of us will want to know about the alternatives to medication. Users want information about the range of services available, particularly on discharge from hospital into the community. This is easy to say and it is easy to agree to, but the action rarely happens. I recently spoke to some people being discharged from a day hospital who didn't know what a community psychiatric nurse is, or that there was a drop in centre 100 yards away. It is crucially important we know our rights, both to receive and refuse treatment.

Choice: everyone is different and not everyone wants the same treatment. Someone who can't sleep may benefit from yoga, sleeping pills, meditation or counselling, but which of these do mental health workers offer? Someone who is freaking out may well welcome an admission to an acute ward, but for someone else it may be what they most fear. Is there a crisis house which relies less on medication, and what about intensive support to stay at home? Above all, time and time again, people say that the choice that is missing is someone to talk to.

On accessibility: service users do want services that are near their homes and we want them to be open when we need them. Mental health crises do not conveniently occur between 9.00 and 5.00, and for us Christmas can be the loneliest time. I'm pleased to hear of the moves that are being made in Glasgow to provide these kind of services. Service users want somewhere other than an Accident and Emergency Department, a place we can simply turn up to and say: "Help, I'm in a mess"; the more hoops that users have to jump through to access a particular service and the longer we have to wait, the more sure you can be that users of that service will be determined more by social status and assertiveness than by need.

On advocacy: generally, service users are scared of mental health workers. Professionals might not feel very intimidating but there's something about the relationship that we have with you, especially if you're a doctor, which means that we're scared of you. Obviously the powers under the Mental Health Act have a lot to do with this. It's not easy for us to say, or even think, what we want in a situation such as a ward round or review, especially if we fear that what we want to say is not what the mental health workers want to hear. Service users need access to independent, funded advocacy services, to support them to put their views across.

Equal opportunities: Service users want a service that takes account of the whole range of attitudes to emotional distress or mental illness. Is it more rational, for example, to believe that there is a mind but not to believe that there's a soul? No-one has the monopoly on the truth when it comes to mental health. We need to recognise that racism and sexism and, dare I say, even Majorism, can drive you mad. People who, for example, are working class or who are mothers, who are perhaps gay or lesbian, want workers who they trust to understand their experiences, and that means fair promotion opportunities in the services for people from a range of different backgrounds, and it means the kind of training for mental health workers that currently they rarely get.

Services need to offer privacy, security and freedom from harassment, from staff and other users. Don't assume that its not an issue in your hospital or mental health project. One study of residents in a psychiatric hospital found that 71% had been threatened with physical violence; 38% had been sexually assaulted and 27% had been sexually assaulted by staff[2]. Certainly I know of a number of day centres in London that have been taken over by men in such a way that women actually feel unable to use that service. In a US study, 15% of male therapists actually admitted to sexual contact with clients, 92% of them women.[3] To give some quotes from some research into the experience of black psychiatric patients in Leicester[4]; from a woman patient: "They would call you names and say you were a mad black woman. There was one nurse and I really didn't like her. She would say how mad all black people are". And from a male patient: "I found the patients even more racist than the staff. One of them had the habit of calling me 'Sambo'. I couldn't believe it - even the mad people hate us. I told the nurse and she told me I was imagining it all". And later talking about the staff: "I became very wary of all the white people and the only black people I saw were the cleaners". Service providers must implement good equal opportunities policies and programmes.

On income and employment: please do close down the big institutions but don't dump us in special needs ghettos where we go to day centres, not to meet their emotional needs but because otherwise we can't afford to eat and to keep ourselves warm. Professionals can't do much about the recession and welfare benefits cutbacks, but they can set up housing and employment schemes that give us some money to spend, and training schemes to give us the skills to compete for jobs: and recognise that we may be able to make positive use of our experiences by working for your mental health services.

On self help: this is not about mental health services on the cheap - it's about unleashing our desires and abilities to support one another, and to come up with new and imaginative solutions. The Hearing Voices Network, is a fine example of this and to quote from their information leaflet. "The network has been set up to assist voice hearers to find their own ways of coming to terms with their voices, by showing that there are various explanations for the experience of hearing voices which have been shown to empower voice hearers, enabling them to live with the experience in a positive way. There are people who find ways of coping with their voices other than the use of drugs and who have found alternative explanations for their voices outside of the psychiatric model, which has assisted people in coping with their voice experience. The knowledge gained by people who can cope with their voices can be beneficially shared. People who hear voices can be assisted in developing ways of coping with their voices by participating in self help groups in which they can share experiences, explanations and methods of coping, and benefit from mutual support. People who hear voices, their families and friends, can gain great benefit from de-stigmatising the experience, leading to greater tolerance and understanding. This can be achieved through promoting more positive explanations, which give people a framework for developing their own ways of coping, and by raising awareness about the experience in society as a whole".[5]

And finally, self organisation: service users have a lot to contribute to the design and implementation of services, but our experience, knowledge and abilities remain locked away unless we have opportunities to meet together, to find common ground, and to think about what we really want and how to go about getting it. For that, properly funded and supported patients' councils, local service users' forums and national networks are needed.

A test of whether professionals are prepared to respond to users demands is to ask whether a professional would ask his employer to pay three hundred pounds to come to a two-day conference organised by Scottish Service Users to put across their vision of a community-based mental health service? And, if so whether they could stand sitting through it for one and half days before they heard from a professional worker? This is the experience of service users at the Scottish Conference.

References

1   Experiencing Psychiatry: Users' Views of Services. Anne Rogers, David Pilgrim and Ron Lacey. Macmillan/MIND, 1993.

2   Nibert D, Copper S, and Crowmaker M (1989). Assaults against residents of a psychiatric institution: residents' history of abuse. Journal of Interpersonal Violence 4 (3) 342-349.

3   Bouhoustos J., Holroyd J, Lerman H, Forer B and Greenberg M (1983) Sexual intimacies between psychotherapists and patients. Professional: Research and Practice. 14 (2), 185-196.

4   Sadness in my Heart: Racism and Mental Health. Leicester Black Mental Health Group, University of Leicester, 1989.

5   Hearing Voices Network, c/o MACC, Swan Buildings, 20 Swan Street, Ancoats, Manchester M4 5JW. Tel: 061-834-9823.

THE CONTRIBUTION OF SERVICE USERS IN THE DESIGN AND IMPLEMENTATION OF SERVICES

LAWRENCE NUGENT

I would like to speak about users empowerment and the enablement of it. From the Glasgow perspective or view, it is unfortunate that the involvement of users is with the higher structures of the Greater Glasgow Health Board, such as the sector managers rather than to the people that the service users need to be in contact with in relation to planning a proper quality of service. The users should be enabled and empowered to be involved in every structure, whether its discussion with the Glasgow Health Council, the voluntary organisations, the statutory organisations or the Greater Glasgow Health Board.

Users need the tools of empowerment; they need full training and that is a long process. Over the last two years, from the first stakeholders meeting, there has been developments at the highest levels to assist the service uses to that end of planning and developing, hopefully, the strategy of the Greater Glasgow Health Board. The users' voice should not only be heard at the stakeholding meetings organised by the Greater Glasgow Health Board but truly involved in consultation and planning of the services and at the highest level they're doing that; unfortunately it's not hitting the street level or community level. I believe that mental health teams should be doing more to assist that process and helping users - particularly with training packages on the particular issues that affect them. This has never been seen as tokenistic by the higher levels and we haven't seen it as tokenistic, the users who have been in these meetings have seen that the people who have involved us in the consultation are genuinely trying to give the users not only a voice but getting their participation in the planning of services at community level and at hospital level.

The real spin-off has been the ongoing enablement by the sector managers to get their teams to help and assist the users to be a working part in the building of this new approach in giving and ensuring a good, ongoing quality health service. A good model of this community care in particular is the North Sector, who took up the challenge at the stakeholding meeting and set out to establish a sector-wide structure that would bring the community mental health team's service closer and more efficiently to people. Lesley Wilson, the North Sector Manager, has encouraged uses and her teams to organise themselves into a consumer-led group that will assist the process of assessment, advocacy and consultation for all. John Blackwood, the Service Manager, with the assistance of the Maryhill Users' Group, is now looking at setting up a patients' council. This is at an advanced stage and only the funding has got to be sorted out. Of course proper space is essential. Please be genuine in your part of helping us, the users, to empowerment and setting up a patients' council and a community network for the users - be realistic, give us space, give us office administration to whatever we need.

We're here - get in touch with us and we will communicate. I've met four professionals and we are trying to set up structures to help - the users and their communities to start looking at setting up organisational structures which can feed into the strategy and planning at a health board level. That's the type of things that we as users want out of this. We want to make contact with people who can help us to our own empowerment, train us to assist you in developing policy, because you may be a user - you probably are users of the services.

THE CONTRIBUTION OF SERVICE USERS IN THE DESIGN AND IMPLEMENTATION OF SERVICES

BRIAN SMITH

I'm on the executive of SUN. Most of you have only heard of one SUN. The SUN I am speaking of is the Scottish Users' Network; a network of users and end-users and user groups of psychiatric services.

In the spring of this year I was elected to the executive of SUN. I am a chronic manic depressive, I think, and I'm now stabilised on Lithium, I know. Before that I could make a light bulb glow in the dark by touching the two terminals. And with that track record I lost my job, I lost my income, I lost my family and I lost my friends. Slowly and slowly family and friends came back, but not job and not income. So today I am on Mr. Lilley's little list -an invalidity benefit scrounger, a poll tax dodger and now a council tax withholder. I count myself a 'disregard', if you know the jargon. Do you know the jargon? Well, if you've got a house with one ordinary person in it he can have a discount, I think, of fifty per cent or something like that. If they have two people - ordinary - then they pay the lot. But if they have one person who is mentally bewildered, he is a 'disregard' and this person gets the exemption whether or not the ordinary person is in the house. Now I live alone as a disregard, so for council tax purposes I don't exist.

When I joined the SUN executive, I learnt of the crippling insult of the Scottish Office - and I am glad to know that there are some Scottish Office people at this conference. In the Year of Community Care established on April Fools' Day 1993, SUN the user network was denied even the meagre funding it had previously enjoyed. The really patronising insult was the gift of a grant of a thousand pounds to commission a fund-raising brochure. I have the draft of it in my hand now. In other words, it's privatising a public service which put user participation into the legislation. So the government enshrines user input into mental health care planning and action and castrates the only emergent body which represents all users in Scotland suffering from whatever mental illness. I hope you will go back to the Scottish office and think on that.

On November 9th I have to take part in a second meeting with HEBS, the Health Education Board for Scotland. At our first meeting they produced an already printed, glossy five year plan - some of you may have seen it, I don't know. I kid you not, mental health had no place in its five priorities. Its five priorities were determined by whether you could quantify them and publish the successful results. The sort of thing was: "we're going to reduce heart attacks by 25%, we're going to cut smoking down by 1%". But mental health you couldn't deal with like that, so it found no place in HEBS priorities. To get there, the cure had to be quantifiable.

I have been asked to bring to this meeting on November 9th my five priorities for health care. I went through the list of attenders at this conference last night and there are no HEBS people today so I can speak with that freedom which courtesy might otherwise deny me. So I'm going to give you the five priorities which I intend to take to HEBs on November 9th and you can shout "Boo" or "Hooray" according to whether you think I've got it right or wrong.

My first priority is money. Money is the great enabler, the great empowerer. Money is the universal medicine for the mentally ill. It is cheap to give and simple to administer. If you are going to put ill or recovering people into the community, you must give them the cash to pay their way. They will pay you back later by reduced demands on an expensive hospital service. Boo or Hooray?

Audience: "Hooray!"

Priority 2: **Continuing support and encouragement.** Now that's a cliché. I have had a monthly visit from a trained psychiatric social worker from my hospital since perhaps 1980. I trust him implicitly. Now if I have an attack I will pull the hospital communication cord - before it was always handcuffs, massive doses of largactyl and hospital 80 miles away in an ambulance. Now I manage my illness. I do not want to see some half-baked but well meaning social worker who knows little about a specialist field and doesn't know me. I have not had a Section and a hospitalisation since 1984 and for me that's an achievement. And that has saved the NHS a lot of money.

I didn't do a "Boo, Hooray" on that. The management of illness by the patient, I think, is something which is achievable but it means that you have to treat the user as a carer and the carer as a user, and you might get somewhere. This describes my relationship with Wilf Hughes, the psychiatric social worker from whom I've gained so much. I care for him.

Priority 3: SUN - **Scottish Users Network.** Yes, I'm angry about the funding cut. It is criminal cynicism to will the end and then refuse the means, and that is what seems to have happened to all the people involved in SUN, and it's making our life very difficult. I'm going to do a little sort of schoolmastery test - put up your hand if you've actually heard of the Scottish Users Network ....oh my goodness, I didn't expect that - I thought three of you might have. OK, now all user services are underfunded, we agree. The individual illness organisations like National Schizophrenia Fellowship, Alzheimers' Society and so on, and the politically correct learning difficulties - I thought they were called Downs Syndromes - they have their own fund-raising and their own priorities but they need a dog with teeth and expertise to deal with hospital managements, health boards, the Scottish Office. I would say that SUN was emergent in that field and Scotland has a little advantage over England in respect that we can look at our country as a whole without being overwhelmed by the mountain that we're looking at.

Priority Number 4: **SUN Link.** None of you have heard of that. It's my baby and it's still in the womb. It has been adopted by the SUN executive, it has had an airing at the first Scottish Association of Mental Health (SAMH) Advisory Council meeting in Stirling last spring. You will find it in Appendix 1 of the SUN brochure which has been commissioned for the thousand pounds. This has reached the proof stage now. So when you get the fundraising brochure, if you come across it, have a look at Appendix 1 SUN Link. Briefly, it is conceived as a monitoring service by users covering the whole mental health field. That is the vision. It contains proposals like users being paid when they do a carer's job - we'll do a "Boo, Hooray" on that one, please.

Audience: "Hooray" Yeah, mm, yes - that will make it happen.

And Priority Number 5 - that bring me full circle to my first and last priority - **money.** Carers have it, users don't. But carers should remember that they could easily become users. And providers get it. If users provide, they should be treated as providers, however small the scale. You pay your babysitter - well, maybe you don't. Right - you should pay your befriender, your advocate, your person who brings experience, comfort and encouragement because he or she has been through the mill. All the members of SUN are people with user experience. If you want to join SUN as a non user then you pay a lot more money and get no vote. If you really want a contribution from service users in the design and implementation of services, and it's not just lip service, you must give what you expect for yourselves - the rate for the job. You might find you save a lot of money, and by restoring their dignity and worth, help heal a lot of hurt people.

COMMUNITY MENTAL HEALTH TEAMS

JOE BOUCH

Introduction

The past thirty years has been a time of great social change. Institutionalism and traditionalism have been challenged in many settings. The health service has not been free of such challenges and particularly the traditional professions of medicine and nursing have had to carefully consider (a) what they do; (b) how they do it; (c) how they might improve it.

The policy of community care has gathered pace and in recent years the needs of those with severe psychiatric illnesses have been highlighted. Cases such as those of Ben Silcock (a man with schizophrenia who climbed into the lions' enclosure in London Zoo and was mauled) and Christopher Clunis (a man with schizophrenia who killed the musician Jonathan Zito) have caused considerable anxiety. It has been argued, particularly in the media, that such cases were a direct result of community care and de-institutionalisation.

Community mental health services must recognise the needs of targeting the severely mentally ill and making their needs the priority of the service. The severely mentally ill are usually psychotic (suffering from both delusions and hallucinations); have major social needs (and are often not in receipt of the benefits to which they are entitled); are often known to many agencies but claimed by none; are sometimes hidden away, withdrawn and too frightened to surface and let their needs be known.

Prioritising the Severely Mentally Ill

	1982/1983 Figures 1000 pop/year
Cases with mental health problems	250-315
GP (90 treated only for physical symptoms)	230
GP recognises as psychiatric morbidity	101.5
GP refers to psychiatric services	20.8
Admitted to psychiatric bed	3.3

Goldberg F. Filters to care - a model In: Indicators for Mental Health in a population Eds. R. Jenkins and S. Griffiths, London: HMSO 1990.

Similar results have been replicated in Holland and Italy. Thus psychiatric services already priorities the most severe mental health problems. A further prioritisation needs to take place however whereby resources are targeted at those with 'persistent severe mental illnesses'.

In my own service in Clydebank there is a population of 48,000 and an identified group of 200 persistently severely mentally ill. This would suggest an annual incidence of between 4 and 5 new cases per year for the area. Clydebank is a small town on the outskirts of Glasgow. There is a mixed population epidemiologically with some semi-rural areas and major areas of severe urban deprivation.

There are many reasons for targeting those with persistent severe mental illness. They are the group who are most at risk from suicide, homelessness, and more occasionally homicide. They represent a severe burden both on carers and on hospital services. They are the least able to demand appropriate services. Finally, good management can make a massive difference to the lives of these patients.

Some of the difficulties demonstrated in the above diagram can be better dealt with by a comprehensive integrated community service. Keyworkers and more experienced clinicians dealing with this group of patients leads to far better continuity. It is recognised however that the dangers of the process of 'upward delegation of responsibility' (Isabel Menzies-Lyth) need to be borne in mind. Problems can be identified early, thus hopefully preventing "relapse". If hospital admission is required, this can often be on a planned basis as the assessment will have taken place prior to rather than during admission. Also improved knowledge of patients can lead to a tailoring of management plans to their particular needs. Early discharge is possible as active follow up will take place in the community and thus medication can be appropriately monitored. If the patient defaults from attendance at clinics, he or she can be contacted at home.

Those with persistent severe mental illnesses may be described as having high needs with low demands. They have a need firstly for structure to their daily life. We are accustomed to thinking of people in a high stress situation "burning out" but the particular danger for this group of patients is having insufficient daily demands leading to a process of "rust out" (Jacqueline Atkinson). A second need is for supportive relationships and lastly a need for help with problems of everyday living.

Two case vignettes will serve to illustrate some of these points.

1.   C.M. is a 22 year old woman. She was sexually abused in childhood. She received poor parenting also and has grown into an immature adult who is extremely impulsive. She is physically attractive and makes boyfriends easily but finds the more mature emotional demands of relationships difficult. When such difficulties arise, even seemingly trivial, she responds by taking overdoses. This has led to multiple hospital admissions. Each individual attempt appears insignificant in terms of real suicidal intent, but due to the number of attempts, she is at high suicidal risk. In the past she has been seen by numerous SHO's and Registrars following overdoses and is subsequently either discharged or offered follow up appoints from which she defaults.

2.	T.O. is a 43 year old man separated from his wife. He has a family background permeated with criminal violence to the point that this has become a way of life for him. He suffers from paranoid schizophrenia and also abuses drugs and alcohol. He has marked impairment of short term memory due to this. He talks openly about both suicidal ideation and violent ideation. When he was visited at home by consultant and community nurse, he greeted them with a tea towel over his arm, concealing a machete. He is reluctant to take prescribed antipsychotic medication.

Style of Service Delivery

1.	**Assertive outreach** - This is the principle whereby if those targeted as being most in need of services do not attend the services, then there will be active attempts to reach them in whatever situation that may be. Non-attendance may be due to general disorganisation but sometimes represents a breakdown in the therapeutic relationship or alternatively the non-establishment of a therapeutic relationship. A small group of patients in Clydebank, most of whom suffer from paranoid schizophrenia, have been reluctant to take up services. In this situation we have often adopted a policy of regular visits, perhaps every one to two months to remind the person that we are still there and that they may wish our help. This has invariably led to an improvement in relationships between clinical staff and the patient and a gradual increase in the use of services.

2.	**Crisis prevention** - This principle was outlined previously whereby life problems which may precipitate acute relapse/psychosocial breakdown are identified early and dealt with. (See Diagram 1).

3.	**The therapeutic relationship** - Many of those with persistent severe mental illnesses have paranoid ideas leading to hostility, suspicion and difficulty in forming trusting relationships. This can be helped by having the same keyworker involved, regular contact and low demands to start with from clinicians. There is a need for the patient to perceive that clinicians are on the same side as him or her. In the users' movement, the term 'empowerment' is used and is relevant to the need for patients to be in control of their own lives as far as possible. It is a common practice in my service, for example to establish patients with schizophrenia on a low dose of depot antipsychotic medication with additional oral antipsychotic medication which can be adjusted by the patient him or herself. This has various benefits both helping the patient to understand their illness and the effects of medication and to feel that they are beginning to have some control over their illness rather than seeing themselves as being at the mercy of clinicians.

Multidisciplinary Team Issues

There is a need for a clear and shared vision which must be established by senior clinicians. Staff who have been used to working in a hospital based service face many challenges in adjusting to working in the community. There may be a radical de-skilling accompanying increasing responsibilities. These responsibilities will be to both individual patients in terms of increased clinical autonomy and to the team itself. There is an issue of "ownership". In the early days of the team, a frequently repeated comment was "what do they want us to do" with the "they" never being clearly defined (possibly "the management"). Clinicians have a "need to give" and most will want to do a good job. Being too prescriptive is a mistake. Clinicians have to become more adept in taking part in discussions involving various disciplines, for example in case conferences. There is also a need for each discipline to understand what the other discipline does in order to facilitate cross-disciplinary referrals whereby the most appropriate member of staff will deal with the patient's needs.

With regard to organisation of the team, "contingency theory" is recognised whereby "there is no such thing as the best organisational structure. What is the best structure is contingent upon the size, purpose, age, location and other characteristics of the organisation". Referral meetings, review meetings, case conferences and joint assessments are all important. Clinical supervision is vital for those doing work on for example sexual abuse, cognitive behavioural work and working with families. A clinical planning team has also been developed to review the service and develop new approaches.

SYSTEMIC ISSUES

In addition to issues within the team, the team itself also relates to many other organisations. Development of good relationships between organisations with mutual benefits is of great importance.

Organisational Relations

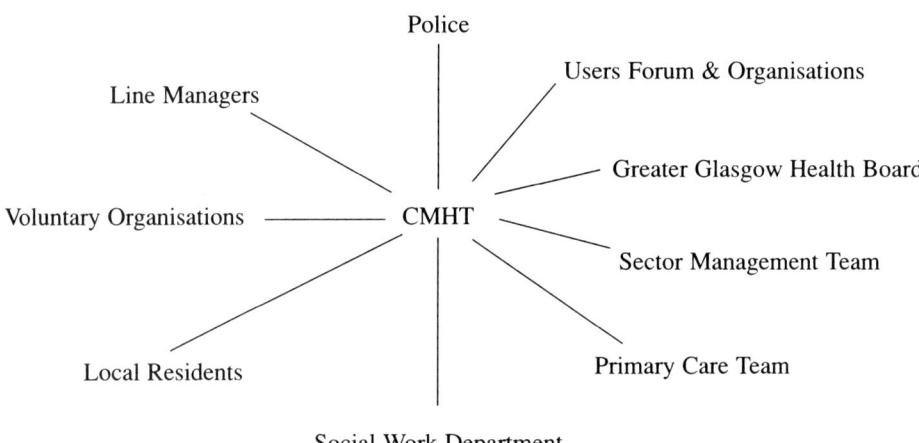

Some Closing Remarks

We have identified some problems that at the moment appear insoluble. There are some patients, for example, who despite our persistence and despite their obvious need, still will not use our service. If mental health services however do not grapple with such problems, then who can be expected to? There may be problems which are insoluble to which there is no obvious answer. We can at least however aim for consensus decisions and do what can be done. Finally tragedies will still happen. It is impossible to eliminate risk although hopefully this can be reduced.

Diagram 1

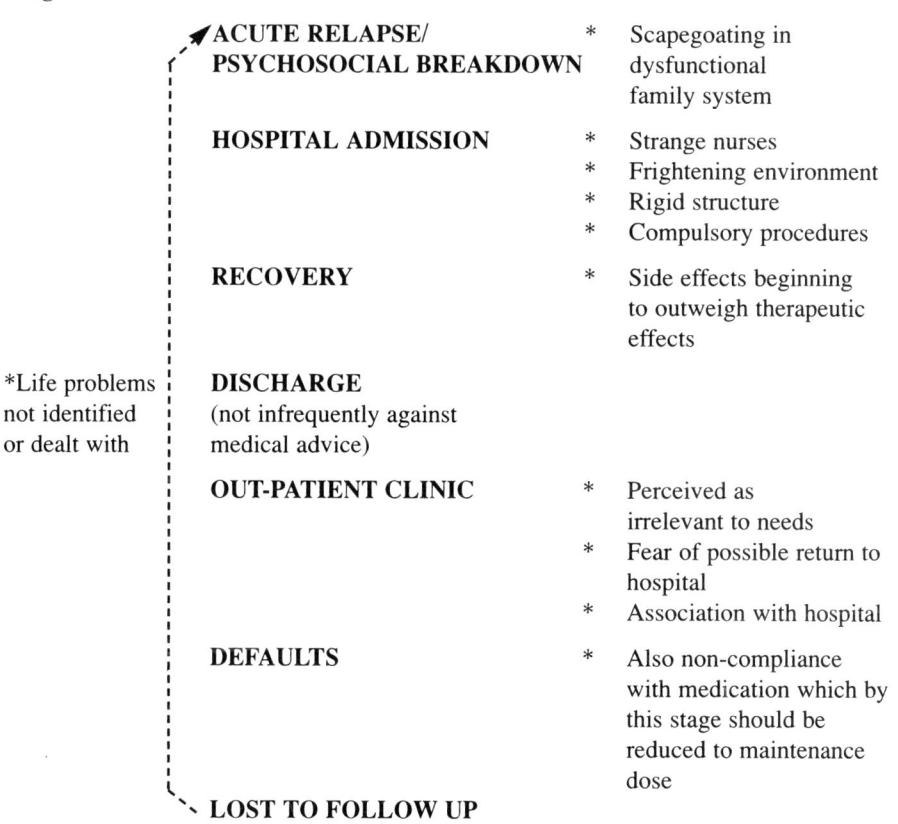

	ACUTE RELAPSE/ PSYCHOSOCIAL BREAKDOWN	* Scapegoating in dysfunctional family system
	HOSPITAL ADMISSION	* Strange nurses * Frightening environment * Rigid structure * Compulsory procedures
	RECOVERY	* Side effects beginning to outweigh therapeutic effects
*Life problems not identified or dealt with	**DISCHARGE** (not infrequently against medical advice)	
	OUT-PATIENT CLINIC	* Perceived as irrelevant to needs * Fear of possible return to hospital * Association with hospital
	DEFAULTS	* Also non-compliance with medication which by this stage should be reduced to maintenance dose
	LOST TO FOLLOW UP	

COMMUNITY MENTAL HEALTH TEAMS

LAURIE DAVIDSON

Introduction

The delivery of mental health services through multi-disciplinary Community Mental Health Teams (CMHTs) was once seen as a radical experiment. The community team model is now well established as the model of preference in many parts of the UK, despite recent challenges and threats. In 1985 there were only 20 CMHTs operating throughout the country; [1] now there are over 500. [2] Developing services are still placing the CMHT at the hub of mental health service delivery.

There have been many changes in the last decade which have effected the focus and nature of CMHTs, and there has been a move away from the "centre" based model towards the CMHT as co-ordinator of a wide range of networked community resources including day care, home support and rapid response services, accommodation, community alternatives to hospital , user groups, advocacy and community inpatient facilities. Strong links have been established with other services and voluntary agencies.

The involvement of users, carers and other stakeholders in planning and developing services has necessitated a revolution in the way services are delivered to include a 24 hour response, respite and other community alternatives to hospital as well as improved practical help with housing and finance. The "full caseload" model of many CMHTs, where each team member is fully occupied with allocated clients and cannot respond fully to unscheduled need does not have the capacity to respond to need and teams have been reorganised around service provider rather than user, need. The latest changes in CMHTs have reversed this emphasis, are as exciting as the initial experiment and although some existing teams are slow to change, new teams have often learned the lessons of weak community services and been set up more appropriately.

Why have multi-disciplinary teams?

The ethos of the multi-disciplinary team has survived in spite of the assaults from care management and GP fundholding. The advantages of this approach are worth protecting and are:-

> **Holistic Assessments.** No one person or profession can claim to have a total all embracing perspective or have every skill required for the range of problems and

situations in mental health. When teams have the necessary routines to allow multi-disciplinary input, there is a greater chance that important aspects of the assessment are not missed.

More Choice for Users. The growth of multi-disciplinary teams has produced a revolution in the range of therapeutic and practical help to users. The development of cognitive/behavioural, humanistic and psychodynamic approaches has been stimulated by the need for more efficient and effective methods of treatment. The range of services for people with long term problems has increased and user involvement has flourished alongside the services now that they are more local.

Cross Fertilisation of Skills and Knowledge. The proximity of professionals from a range of training backgrounds and perspectives has enlarged the knowledge base of all team members. While some skills remain unique or specialist, others have become generic and more accessible. Joint working has broken down many stereotypes and prejudices which have plagued mental health services to the detriment of the user.

Ease of Cross Referral. Different professionals and team members are more likely to be accessible in a common team base, and there is more likelihood that the user will get the most appropriate worker rather than Hobson's choice. Specialist skills within the team can be accessed without referring over totally.

Better co-ordinated services. Prime worker responsibility has replaced the fragmented services of the past. In developed CMHTs, the key worker responsibility follows the user wherever they are in the service (including the acute unit) and this improves continuity of care. Locality planning and local stakeholder consultation have begun to generate more appropriate services as a network of statutory, voluntary and ordinary community services. Teams have a higher investment in a defined geographical area where resources are well known and relationships with other teams developed.

Problems with CMHTs

The above picture is a rosy one. Unfortunately, the above advantages are by no means guaranteed, and the reality is that the first generation of CMHTs have made many mistakes along the way.

Lack of User Consultation. Services were set up with professionals in mind. 9 - 5, five day week services were offered. Clinical teams were set up with token skill mixes rather than being led by real demand. When the user was consulted, it was often discovered that the new services fell well short of what was needed to prevent unnecessary or inappropriate admissions, that the staff were often elitist and not prepared to be involved in practical tests and that the service had no alternatives to home or hospital. Users were still angry, and very little had really changed.

Hearing the user voice has resulted in CMHTs - Mark II, evolutionary model based more on the actual needs of users. Services in Sparkbrook, St Albans, Newton Abbot and Glasgow are examples of this new, prioritised approach.

Lack of Targeting. The research of Patmore and Weaver [3] and Liz Sayce [1] confirmed the fear that CMHTs had opened their doors too widely in pursuing open access policies. Efforts to win over local GPs were often too successful, leading to a flood of referrals for depression, anxiety and stress. Although most of these referrals were of people in real distress and were cruelly caricatured as the "unhappy well", those with long term problems were being pushed out by the sheer volume of referrals.

Unmanaged Teams. There was initially a trend towards appointing co-ordinators of CMHTs rather than managers in order to side-step the thorny issues of multi-disciplinary team management. Democracy is laudable, but this style of organisation was often divorced from the wider management structure, had no teeth and no authority or credibility. Co-ordinators often rotated and were appointed regardless of their ability to do the job. Nobody maintained an overview of team activity or was in a position to carry out effective workload management. Professionals became too autonomous and often chose the work that interested them rather than responding to agreed targeting criteria.

Multi-disciplinary problems. Unmanaged teams often found themselves unable to resolve basic rivalries and differences between disciplines and retreated into a seige mentality where caseloads were shrouded in mystery and suspicion and joint working was sometimes seen as admitting failure. The key worker model often meant the user had the skills of one team member rather than the whole team. In this situation, the benefits and "raison d'etre" of the multi-disciplinary team were lost, and working in a team was often unsafe and unpleasant.

Poor Continuity of Care. The relief of moving out of the institution into the community was so strong for some team members that they rarely darkened the hospital doors again. Rivalry sometimes developed between the hospital and community teams with the former accusing the latter of neglecting those in most serious need and of "handing over" problems, conveniently picking them up on discharge when all the real work had been done. The community looked with disdain on the hospital, sometimes directing high-minded criticism at the institution. The user, in the meantime, experienced being handed over between elements of the service with very little continuity, often having to tell their story all over again. On discharge, communication was often poor with a real risk of the user being lost to the service at their most vulnerable time.

Lack of evaluation. Lack of clinical awareness or interest from senior management was often the reason for ill-defined outcome measures. Teams often assumed they were effective and the lack of team management could mean that workers defined their own criteria of success. There was little solid evidence that people's quality of life had improved or that community teams had any effect on admissions or compulsory orders. Evidence that the service had improved was often forthcoming, but was mainly anecdotal and did not do enough to convince the cynic that CMHTs were a good idea.

Poor crisis response. The "full caseload" syndrome of many teams made a full and proper crisis response rare. Although teams often had "on call" systems for emergencies, these often meant that one person carried responsibility for one day only, with problems of continuity and level of commitment. If follow up was offered out of hours, this was often limited to crisis intervention or crisis management rather than the intensive involvement often needed at these times.

Challenges for Community Mental Health Teams

GP Fundholding. The movement from block contracts for mental health services to contracts which may involve a single constituent member of the CMHT is potentially very destructive to the multi-disciplinary team which has not, so far, had to cope with internal competition for work. If, for example, the Psychologist or CPN are purchased by name outside of the team referral process, the team approach itself is threatened. Although there are strong indications from the Department of Health that CPNs should be a secondary care resource, there is nothing to stop fundholding GPs from paying for CPNs from their own budget. In view of the fact that GPs mainly refer people with problems of anxiety and depression, there is a real danger that the secondary care resource will become depleted, disadvantaging those who are a higher priority for the health and social services purchasers and providers.

There are many parallel developments which are strengthening the role of primary care teams such as the employment of counsellors and practice nurses. The work of Rachel Jenkins raises many important questions and a few solutions to the dilemmas of primary care and mental health [4]. It is certainly very important for teams to forge stronger links with primary health care teams generally, not just those which are fundholding.

Care Management.

Can be a threat or an opportunity. Original fears that care management would replace the multi-disciplinary team do not seem to have materialised. The process is either carried out from outside of teams in which case a multi-disciplinary assessment is often commissioned, or team members, or indeed the whole team have been designated care managers in which case it is often business as normal. The value of care management for teams is in accessing devolved budgets, having an advocacy role and tightening up the processes of assessment and review.

Where teams have successfully combined the two models of care management and multi-disciplinary team work, care management is an asset. Where it has resulted in role confusion, care managers not being allowed access to the teams or no change, care management has been less than helpful for the user. The challenge of combining the best of both models is a continuing challenge for managers and teams.

Market Forces. The market could force purchasers to seek lower cost options for mental health services such as enhanced primary health care teams or wider purchasers could regard mental health services as 'less lucrative' in terms of attracting business from outside of the Trust (most people with mental health problems are not likely to travel great distances for better treatment). Cheaper and less local options could start the move back to central resources. Some services might see the Mental Illness Specific Grant as 'taking care' of their obligation to develop better services. Only a major commitment and investment in community services will produce the standard of service demanded by stakeholders.

Targeting problems. With the backlash against the tendency of CMHTs to 'drift' towards the 'unhappy well' the 'walking wounded' and 'new clientele', a false dichotomy has developed between those who are seen as deserving or not. The truth is that the dividing line is not as easy to define, and those with serious mental health problems could end up receiving no service as a result of simplistic constructs. Many different criteria are being applied such as, history, diagnosis, need, problem, distress, treatability and any combination of the aforementioned. The reality is that gatekeeping is a total package which must guide every routine of the multi-disciplinary team process. Teams who have to struggle with the demands of everyday referral bombardment need to have agreed criteria which are responsive to local demand whilst ensuring that those with the greatest need have the biggest slice of the cake.

The most helpful way of prioritising is probably in terms of the management of team resources. The first two groups of clients who should be ring-fenced and given the best possible service are those with long term mental health problems and those who are at risk of hospitalisation or are a danger to self or others. The third group are those who do not fall in the first categories, but who nevertheless present with serious mental health problems. Many of these people will be in severe distress and are not 'unhappy well'. The service given to this group will depend on resources and local assessed need.

Efficiency and effectiveness in CMHTs

There are measures of efficiency in CMHTs which have become clearer over the first decade of community team development. The effective and efficient team will have the following in place:-

Effective team management. There is a need for a team manager who is fully part of the management structure and recognised by both health and social service management.The manager needs to have an overview of all the activity of the team, have access to resources, be given sufficient status within the team to be able to make decisions and carry them through and give a vision and direction to the team. Although it may be possible to jointly manage teams through separate health and social services managers, this relies too heavily on the personalities involved and the joint approach of both agencies. The fully managed team or the team with a designated manager who deals with the day to day management but consults or defers on inter-professional issues seem to hold most chance of success.

Continuity of Care. There is a much used term, but for a modern CMHT it means:-

Retaining prime worker responsibility wherever the user is in the systems, a 'one team approach' between the CMHT and the inpatient unit team, with flexible working boundaries, a combined care planning (care management, care programme approach or, in future, supervised discharge) process between hospital and community, regular review of all high priority clients which includes contingency plans agreed with users and carers, involvement of all specialist assessors e.g., Occupational Therapist, Psychologist, Art Therapist etc. discharge of legal and good practice obligations, Joint record keeping and central files for efficient communication and good relationships with in-patient teams, primary health care teams, social services, linked psychiatric teams and community resources.

Effective rapid response. The team needs to consume its own smoke as far as possible. Risk taking is about knowing the user, the user knowing and trusting the team, good knowledge of local resources, a range of community alternatives to hospital, worker trust of each other and the commitment of all parts of the service including general practitioners (GPs) and junior doctors. Having a crisis management response is not going to produce the desired outcomes of:- preventing unnecessary or inappropriate admissions, shortening the length of in-patient stay, more clarity about the purpose of appropriate admissions and more effective in-patient treatment. What is needed is a total approach to urgent need which includes prevention rather than fire-fighting.

Built-in quality. A range of quality assurance measures are needed for teams to function well: Management, clinical and professional supervision as well as specialist clinical supervision in the practice of some psychotherapy, a variety of audit procedures on file, systems, clinical protocols, reception for users, treatment approaches etc, user involvement and feedback at every level through questionnaires, stakeholders meetings, inspection of services, planning, advocacy, user groups and standard setting, standard setting as prescribed by purchasers and negotiated at team level and inscribed in live operational policies, regular needs assessment with the community. Workload management to ensure priorities are being met, staff are not becoming burnt-out and that the team manager has an overview of all team activity. Regular team reviews, effective business meetings, proper agenda and minute taking practice and effective clinical meetings which make full use of the multi-disciplinary team and research, training and ongoing evaluation.

Multi-Worker model. The key worker approach often came to mean one-to-one involvement with users regardless of whether the key worker had all the necessary skills, knowledge or training. This Hobson's Choice model may be appropriate for straightforward counselling or psychotherapy, but is bad news for people with more complex needs who need access to a variety of resources within the team.

The new, improved CMHT will find ways of ensuring that all the skills of the multi-disciplinary team, other teams and community resources are being accessed on behalf of the user. This involves establishing an ethos of multi-worker involvement which cuts across the one-to-one model and involves joint working, professional-specific pieces of work and a true care package taking a wider perspective than the resources of the team itself.

User responsive. The effective team will find ways of empowering users of the service and their carers which are more than just token. Once again, there is a need for a team ethos which moves away from the purely professional or clinical and takes on a practical and user-friendly image. If service planners and teams listen to users, the way forward will present itself.

Conclusion

The future of community mental health teams is partly in their own hands. If they become effective and efficient, the results will speak for themselves. Those who have grown up professionally in CMHTs may find it hard to believe that such an adaptable model could be supplanted. There are, however, wider trends which threaten the very existence of true multi-disciplinary teams. They may be attractive in the short term, but if they bring about the demise of the multi-disciplinary CMHT, the longer term effects could lead to depleted secondary care services, less choice for the user and the re-emergence of interdisciplinary rivalries.

References

1. Sayce. L., Field V. 'Community Mental Health Centres in the UK' NURDP 1990.

2. Onyett Steve. Informal feedback from initial research soundings on CMHTs.

3. Patmore. C., Weaver T. 'Community Mental Health Teams; lessons for Planners and Managers'. Good Practices in Mental Health 1991.

4. Sayce. L., Craig. T., Boardman. A. 'The Development of Community Mental Health Centres in the UK'. Social Psychiatry and Psychiatric Epidemiology, 26: 14-24 1991.

5. Jenkins. R. 'Developments in the Primary Care of Mental Illness - a Forward Look'. International Review of Psychiatry (1992) 4, 237-242

Also

Jenkins. R., Newton. J., Young R. (Eds) 'The Prevention of Depression and Anxiety - The Role of the Primary Care Team'. HMSO 1992.

ACUTE MENTAL ILLNESS SERVICES

JOHN LOUDON

Dr. John Loudon, spoke as Clinical Director of the Acute Services for Edinburgh. The purpose of the service is to provide comprehensive management of mental disorder as close to the patients home as possible. The total population within the 16-65 year age range served is 286,000.

The directorate is now one year old and combines -

i   Acute Services

ii   The Rehabilitation and Continuing Care Service.

iii   Clinical functions of the University Department of Psychiatry, and MRC Unit for Studies in Brain Metabolism.

iv   A service for tertiary referrals to Scotland.

There are 4 acute sectors with 63,000-82,000 in each sector. Over fifteen per cent of the population are covered by fundholding GPs.

Diagram 1 (Structure of the Acute Service) highlights the relationship of various components of the overall service to the mentally disordered as envisaged by Dr. Loudon. Each component of the diagram has a distinct gap from its neighbour depicting the existence of boundaries. There is a tendency for extra effort to be required for a referral to cross the relevant boundary, and for the more difficult patient to be refused. This happens especially when the team on each side of the boundary is managed separately or has a different employer. Ideally, the future service would contain no boundaries, having a "seamless" systems of care and all providing organisations would be geared towards that goal. Interim goals are to ensure that transfer across the existing gaps are as trouble free as possible. To succeed in this, everyone participating in the overall service must sign up to common aims through the joint planning mechanism. Referral forms and information systems used in common would help enormously.

Dr. Loudon summarised the activity in Edinburgh and the change of direction away from inpatient care over the past 20 years as follows:-

a)   Both acute and continuing care bed numbers have fallen but Day Hospital places, and out-patient clinics in Primary Care settings have increased (Table 1).

b)   In the acute wards bed occupancy runs between 100-115%. The average length of stay has risen over time (now at 35 days). This has occurred in parallel with other developments, including the development of individual care plans prepared by consultation, a shift to continued care provision by other partner agencies (who do not cope with the most needy patients) and some social dislocation. It is a phenomenon found in other urban psychiatric services. Of all admissions, a quarter are compulsory.

c) Since 1974 there have been four sector teams covering the Edinburgh area and since 1990 their boundaries have been coterminous with Social Work districts. The CPN cover equates to one per 30,000 of the population. The Clinical Psychology service is within another directorate and is so resourced that the waiting list currently is eight months.

d) The Emergency Duty Team works throughout the 24 hour period and has a policy of dual assessment by a doctor and a nurse. It provides time limited outreach contact, and liaises with the poisoning treatment ward at the Royal Infirmary.

e) The service feels itself to be fortunate in having close and cooperative working relationships with a number of local authority and SMIG (Specific Mental Illness Grant) funded health projects, housing agencies and voluntary bodies.

f) The service sponsors user feedback and advocacy. The information received has been most helpful in auditing services.

A SWOT analysis of the service, shows in summary:

1   Strengths:

- A start to user involvement,
- user feedback,
- the development of a healthy clinical audit process,
- well developed liaison with other agencies,
- a computerised patient information system,
- a high quality multi-disciplinary work force.

2   Weaknesses:

- Concentration of services in Morningside round the hospital,
- low expenditure on building and decor,
- low quality ward environment as a result of high occupancy.

3   Opportunities:

- A move to sectorised, local, day hospitals,
- the strengthening of clinical initiatives through the directorate,

- local ownership by sector teams of the clinical process,

- resources used to the best advantage.

4   Threats:

- Thrombosis in the acute wards,

- any stand off between Health Social Work and voluntary agencies resulting from resource constraints resulting in service gaps,

- a shift of resources to primary care,

- impoverishing care for the chronically mentally ill.

Diagram 1

STRUCTURE OF THE ACUTE SERVICE

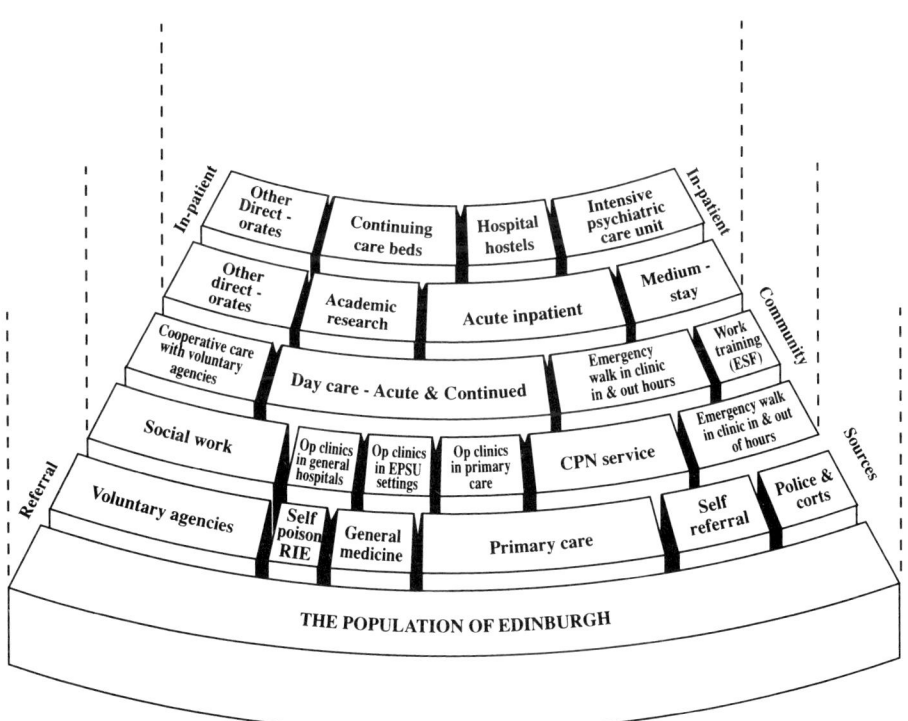

TABLE 1

GENERAL DIRECTORATE - SERVICE DEVELOPMENT

		1973	1983	1993
Outpatient Clinics in Primary				
Care Setting		2	7	10
General Hospitals		3	3	5
Day Hospital places	Acute	-	30}	119
	Rehabilitation	60	60}	
Acute bed numbers		172	99	99
Academic and Research bed numbers		74	74	43
Medium Stay Unit		-	30	15
Continuing Care beds		260	192	103
Hospital Hostels		40	40	52

SERVICES FOR GROWTH AND DEVELOPMENT - THE RIGHT TO BE ORDINARY

NIGEL HENDERSON

The "right to be ordinary" is the challenge when providing services for growth and development. Enabling people with long term mental health problems to lead ordinary, comfortable lives as citizens in the community should be the aim, particularly as many people will have experienced lives that have been anything but ordinary - in fact their lives have been extra-ordinary.

The three main obstacles to providing services that enable personal growth and development are.

1. **The people who provide services** often have to work in a way that does not provide an enabling or empowering relationship to be developed. With the introduction of the Community Care Act they have been bombarded with terms such as monitoring, inspection, reviews, cost management, financial assessment, performance indicators etc. etc. There is a considerable risk that the individual needs of people are lost within the very system that is supposed to meet their needs.

   Do service providers encourage people to challenge themselves and to take risks or do they simply try to meet the basic needs of food, warmth and shelter because, resources and time are finite?

2. **The people who receive services** often feel devalued or unworthy. Many also experience apathy and lack of motivation. It can be very challenging trying to offer services that are meaningful if the service users don't participate as fully as the providers would like.

3. **The people who live near services** are included as an obstacle because more projects are experiencing the NIMBY (not in my back yard) syndrome.

Perhaps to view these three groups of people as obstacles rather than champions for services for growth and development is unduly pessimistic. This could be because providers have been conditioned by a system that constantly highlights the problems and difficulties rather than looking at, and working with, the positive aspects.

How do we accentuate the positive? How do we enable people to feel valued and worthwhile? How do we replace community fears with acceptance?

Penumbra tries to offer an ordinary life to people with long term mental health problems. It offers people supported accommodation in ordinary housing. Until the introduction of the Community Care Act people were offered permanent accommodation. That choice has been eroded by the Act as people can only stay as long as their social work assessment dictates and many of Penumbra's tenants had to be reassured that they could stay after 1 April 1993. Security of tenure was previously something that the tenants valued highly when asked what they like about Penumbra.

Penumbra does not have offices in its houses or keep day to day records on people. Instead each house has a small team of staff which provides the support required by building good relationships and understanding with tenants. Whilst each house works to a common philosophy, the reality is that they all have their own styles of living. In some of the houses tenants are fiercely house proud whilst in others the staff have to encourage people to participate in domestic chores - just as in many ordinary family houses.

Penumbra tenants are mainly people who have spent a considerable number of years in psychiatric hospitals. When asked what the main differences are between hospital and Penumbra most people said that they have more freedom in Penumbra. Privacy was also highly rated, as every tenant has their own lockable room. Many tenants also commented that they did not feel under pressure to change or to do things in a certain "acceptable" way1. This is consistent with Penumbra's philosophy of "accepting people as they are". Penumbra does not set out to provide rehabilitation or therapy. Very simply we attempt to offer an "ordinary home". This is achieved by providing appropriate emotional and practical support.

Penumbra staff work alongside, and with, tenants, they do not do things to, or for, people. Often the outcome of this approach is that people grow and develop at their own pace and in a way that meets the lifestyle they have chosen for themselves.

To enable the development of services that embrace "the right to be ordinary", the following challenges should be considered.

Services have to be meaningful to the consumer. Many consumers feel unclear about the benefits of some of the services they receive. In particular, I am thinking of a number of people who were asked to attend day hospitals once they had been discharged to supported accommodation. They felt that the hospital wanted to "keep an eye on them" and that there were no immediate benefits to them. The result was that they stopped going and were ultimately discharged from the day hospital.

More innovation and experimentation is required. There is a danger that the services provided in the community become very tightly prescribed by the introduction of the purchaser/provider split. As more and more "standards" are introduced it becomes more difficult for providers to offer services that reflect different philosophies. More pilot projects should be funded and research and evaluation included as an integral part of these projects.

Projects offering personally challenging experiences should be developed. A recent trip to Brittany in France with 5 of Penumbra's tenants for a two-week holiday highlighted how little is on offer to people with long term mental health problems by way of personally challenging experiences. People with long term mental health problems should have the opportunity to try outward bound activities in a safe and supported situation. Offering people opportunities that expand horizons and experiences should be a fundamental part of enabling people to develop themselves, instead of it often being considered a luxury.

Services users need to make their voices heard. Providing services that offer opportunities for growth and development will not happen in a meaningful way if the service users are not involved. Training, guidance, support and financing need to be provided to ensure that service users can develop ways of representing their views. They also need to know that their views are taken seriously. Independent advocacy services should be more widely available.

Services should be ordinary. Services should not stand out in the community. This is now widely accepted. The challenge is how to make services people centred. This would include moving away from a clinical continuum which is often problem orientated. Like other citizens, people with mental health problems should not have their needs exclusively determined by health or ill-health.

Self worth and self esteem should be encouraged. Too many people with long term mental health problems feel unworthy or lack confidence. Whilst this can, to a certain extent, be attributed to the long term effects of mental illness, it is not the whole picture.

Too many services still do not enable people to make real or meaningful decisions. If people are to grow and develop personally, they need to be supported to make decisions and mistakes and then to learn from the experience.

REFERENCE

1. Petch Alison, "Heaven compared to a hospital ward". Social Work Research Centre, Stirling University, 1990. ISBN No. 0901636 975

SERVICES FOR GROWTH AND DEVELOPMENT - RESIDENTIAL CARE FOR PEOPLE WITH SEVERE AND PERSISTENT MENTAL HEALTH PROBLEMS

ISOBEL MORRIS

Introduction

The types of residential care settings which were developed in the 1960s and 1970s tended to provide relatively low support. Although assistance could be given with the activities of daily living the level of support and expertise available did not offer a community alternative to people with the most severe mental health problems who continued to be cared for in the large psychiatric hospitals. Therefore, one of the challenges of hospital closure programmes has been to develop innovative residential settings for those most handicapped by mental health problems. This paper describes residential projects developed in Lewisham and North Southwark by the Guy's and St Thomas Trust for this group of people.

If new community based services are to effectively replace the mental hospitals, the needs of 2 groups of patients have to be considered. People who continue to reside in mental hospitals are described in a number of studies (Clifford et al 1991; O'Driscoll et al 1993) as being very elderly and highly dependent. Many had spent the bulk of their adult lives in mental hospitals and their major mental health problems had been compounded by the effects of institutionalisation. If mental hospitals are to close the needs of this group of people must be met in the community. The considerable investment in new facilities required to accommodate them must also meet the needs of future generations of people with severe mental health problems who have not shared the experience of lengthy periods of life in the institution. Their needs and aspirations are likely to be different from those of the very institutionalised population. We tried to solve this problem, not entirely successfully, in ways which I will describe.

What are the problems which challenge us?

The characteristics of the population to be resettled are summarised in table 1. Existing provision in the community prior to the closure programme was largely low staffed and could not meet the needs of this highly vulnerable group of people. Forty per cent of residential accommodation was low support with a maximum of once weekly visits by staff. Twenty two per cent of accommodation provided daily support but not 24 hour care and 32% of places were in 24 hour care facilities. However, the 24 hour support settings all offered medium term rehabilitation with an expectation that residents would move on. No high support was available in permanent homes with no expectation of moving on. The emphasis on the development of new facilities was therefore on this type of accommodation.

Only one setting in the reprovision programme did not provide 24 hour care, although it does provide daily support. A second setting was designed for active elderly people who require 24 hour care but do not present with major behavioural problems. The average length of stay of this group was 48 years. Despite this they have adapted to life in the community, been on holiday several times and report satisfaction with their new home in the community. Two settings provide high support for people who still experience very poorly controlled symptomatology and at times are behaviourally disordered. In these settings it is necessary to combine good quality social care with the expertise and confidence traditionally available in hospitals. Finally, 2 DOMUSES were developed. These are small nursing homes (12 beds) for people who are highly dependent and can be behaviourally disturbed. This is a model of care pioneered in Lewisham and North Southwark by Professor Elaine Murphy and Dr Alistair McDonald Consultants in our service for elderly people with mental health problems. These registered nursing homes are homely environments for elderly people, with high dependency needs to enable them to spend their final years in a dignified way, despite severe and deteriorating cognitive and emotional impairment.

Outcome

The new residential facilities were evaluated by RDP (Pickard et al 1992). During the resettlement programme 59 people were resettled back into our local community. Eight people died between the RDP survey in 1988 and the closure of the hospital in 1991. Only one man with very severe behavioural disturbance resulting from an autistic condition moved to another hospital, a private specialist facility. During the course of the reprovision programme 6 people had readmissions to acute psychiatric wards. However, on the whole the residential settings managed to continue to support residents at home despite fluctuations in mental state and behaviour. Two people were readmitted and remained in another mental hospital which the District uses for longer than one year. Being an elderly population, deaths were monitored before and after the move to the community. There was no evidence of increased mortality as a result of the reprovision programme. Between the Research & Development in Psychiatry (RDP) survey in 1988 and the closure of the hospital in 1991 eight people died in hospital prior to being resettled in the community. Of those resettled five died in their new homes over the same period of time. This included one patient who committed suicide after one year in the community. No patients were lost to the service through drift into vagrancy. (Table 3). In 2 out of 3 homes evaluated following the reprovision the social functioning of the residents improved. Interestingly this was particularly marked in one of the Domuses with people who had very severe impairments of social functioning. There was no change in ratings of behavioural disturbance. The move to the community did not therefore unsettle the patients in a way which resulted in an exacerbation of their disturbance. These results are published in detail in the final RDP Report, Evaluating the Closure of Cane Hill Hospital (Pickard et al 1992).

The RDP research team also investigated the views of residents who moved into the new facilities. Prior to resettlement forty-six percent had not wished to leave hospital. Despite this once settled into their new homes 64% did not wish to return to hospital; seventy-one percent reported liking their new home and eighty-nine percent either liked their new home or felt ambivalent. On the whole most residents could identify improvements in their life though there were aspects of hospital life which they missed. Some residents found the expectations of them in their new homes to be too high. One resident in the non 24 hour care homes mentioned that she missed everything being done for her as had happened in hospital. In giving patients more opportunities for independence in the community we must be careful not to overburden them in a way which is detrimental to their quality of life. Other patients missed the network of social relationships which had been present in the hospital. Although mental hospital can seem bleak to the outside observer, often a subtle network of relationships exists in the wards and the corridors which is not a feature of the strees of Inner London. Interestingly it is some of the more able patients who had developed a satisfying niche for themselves in the hospital who found the change most difficult.

New Facilities and Future Generations

It was mentioned earlier that the reprovision programme represented a major investment in community mental health services but how relevant would the new facilities be to future generations of younger people with severe and persistent mental health problems? Profiles of younger new long stay patients who are accumulating in the mental hospitals suggest that they are less dependent, physical problems are less prominent but symptomatology is poorly controlled and behavioural problems are potentially challenging to manage in the community (Mental Health Unit, Guy's and St Thomas Trust 1992). It was anticipated that the 2 high support homes would be relevant to the needs of our new long stay population. However, the homes have not proved to be appropriate for younger people who have not shared the experience of long term hospitalisation. Nevertheless there are some patients without the experience of long-term hospitalisation who appreciate more communal living and have benefitted from placement in the high support homes. Some of this group had not coped in less supported community settings and would have joined the ranks of the mental hospital population had the high support facility not been available.

However, one third of new long stay patients accumulating in Lewisham and North Southwark are people over 50 who have become severely ill late in life. In addition, there is an increasing population of elderly people over 85 who will need nursing home care as a result of progressive organic conditions. There is therefore evidence that facilities developed for the elderly will continue to have an important role. The 2 Domuses developed for elderly people with high dependency needs and functional mental illness will in future meet the needs of elderly people in our district suffering from progressive dementia. High dependency places will also be available in these settings for younger people with progressive organic conditions. The unit developed for the active elderly is designed as individual bedsits with communal accommodation. Although the initial residents prefer to live communally due to their long experience of living together in hospital, future residents might prefer to have more autonomy. Already this flexibility is proving useful and 2 residents have moved from one of our high support houses to this home because they were interested in more space and privacy than their supported housing provides.

Conclusion

The reprovision programme has been encouraging, demonstrating that within an inner city district it is possible to develop an alternative service to mental hospital care. Results have been positive indicating that even very elderly people with a lengthy experience of institutional life can enjoy new opportunities available to them less distanced from others in their community. Problems have not been experienced with the local community. Neighbours, local shopkeepers and churchgoers have been interested and supportive. We have found that the local community in inner London has been more accepting and good hearted than the media would usually have us believe!

References

Clifford P, Charman A and Webb Y and Best S (1991)

Planning for Community Care: long-stay populations of hospitals scheduled for rundown or closure. British Journal of Psychiatry, 158, 190-196.

O'Driscoll C, Wills W, Leff J, Margolious O (1993)

The TAPS Project 10: The long-stay populations of Friern and Claybury Hospitals: The baseline survey. In, Evaluating the transfer of care from psychiatric hospitals to district based services. (Ed J Leff) British Journal of Psychiatry 162, Supplement 19, 30-35.

Pickard L, Proudfoot R, Woolfson P, Clifford P, Holloway F and Lindsely J (1992).

Evaluating the Closure of Cane Hill Hospital, RDP, London.

The Mental Health Unit , Guy's and St Thomas' Trust (1992)

Lewisham and North Southwark Patients in Bexley Hospital. Report of a Survey Carried out Between October and December 1991.

TABLE 1

Lewisham and North Southwark Patients in Cane Hill
(Data from RDP Survey 1988)

Number	67
Mean Age	66.6 years (range 32.3 - 92.3 years)
% >60	72.4
Mean length of stay	29.4 years (range 2.3 - 62.5 years)
Percentage new long-stay	9.1
% poor/very poor social functioning	40.9
% severe behavioural problems	33.3
% significant physical disability	34.8
% incontinent	18.2

TABLE 2

The New Facilities

Facility	Staff Cover	Night Cover	Staff Ratio	Day shift
FWA	Day time only (unreg)	None	2:5/6 0.3:1	1
St James	24 hour (reg care home)	Sleep in	9:7 1.3:1	2:1:1
Dunton Road	24 hour (reg care home)	2 waking	13:8 1.6:1	2/3
Brandon House	24 hour (reg care home)	1 waking 1 sleeping	14:8 1.7:1	3
Cordwell Road	24 hour (nursing home)	Waking	21:12 1.7:1	4
Dillwyn	24 hour (nursing home)	Waking	21:12 1.7:1	4

TABLE 3

Number	67	
Deaths before leaving hospital (1988-1991)	8	12%
Deaths after leaving hospital (1988-1991)	5	8%
Resettled in the community	58	98%
Transferred to private hospital	1	2%
Brief readmissions	4	7%
Readmissions > 1 year	2	4%
Lost from care	0	

SERVICES FOR GROWTH AND DEVELOPMENT - COMMUNITY CARE FOR PEOPLE WITH PERSISTENT AND LONG-TERM MENTAL HEALTH NEEDS IN PRIVATE HOMES

JERRY BEREIKA

An array of services are required to assist people in developing the skills and environmental supports to become successful and satisfied in their living, learning and working environment, thereby achieving full community integration and presence (Anthony, 1989). There are several key concepts in this statement. Services should:

- involve a practical and functional orientation on skills and environmental supports.

- involve working towards goals of consumer success and satisfaction, the latter all too often forgotten in many service schemes.

- include a multi-dimensional focus on all the major areas of a person's life.

- focus less on treating the person as psychopathology, and more on helping to improve the person's relationship to his or her social-cultural-economic environment.

Several diverse areas of the literature yield a convergence of themes that can guide providers in developing services to maximise community support and integration. Relevant segments of the literature include those which focus on psychiatric rehabilitation theory and practice, supported housing schemes, mental health consumer advocacy, and consumer preferences and satisfaction.

First, important and relevant themes run throughout the **psychiatric rehabilitation literature** espoused by Anthony and others (Anthony, 1979; Cohen, 1989; Anthony et al., 1990; Campenelli et al., 1992). (see Table 1).

TABLE 1

MAJOR THEMES OF THE PSYCHIATRIC REHABILITATION LITERATURE

- Consumer empowerment, participation and choice.

- Individualised, client centred service planning with a focus on consumer goals and preferences.
- An emphasis on improving skill competencies.
- Flexible, eclectic services and supports that change with the needs of the individual.

Similar themes emerge from the literature on the <u>supported housing movement</u>, perhaps most prominently expressed by Carling, among others (Carling et al., 1987; Blanch et al., 1988; Carling, 1990; Brown and Wheeler, 1990; Livingstone et al., 1992). (see Table 2).

TABLE 2

MAJOR THEMES OF THE SUPPORTED HOUSING LITERATURE

- Consumer self-determination.

- Client-centred service planning.

- Meeting basic needs for stable and normal housing, income and social relationships.

- Flexible, individualised and comprehensive supports provided to people in their accommodation settings.

- Focus on full community integration and participation.

There is an emerging literature on what has been referred to as **"individualised" services or "wrap-around" services.** The term "wrap-around" has been most utilised in the children's service sector, but it is likely to find more common usage in the adult sector, as well. In general terms, it refers to the practice of "wrapping" individualised supports and services around a person to meet his or her unique needs at a particular time. It requires considerable flexibility and responsiveness and a willingness to provide or arrange services that do not fall within a traditional definition of mental health care.

This section of the literature provides additional support for the themes already reviewed, particularly in terms of client-centred services, but some new themes also emerge. (see Table 3). Practitioners of this approach (Burchard & Clark, 1990, VanDen Berg, 1993) also emphasize the provision of unconditional care and support, outcome measurement, and flexible funding to support service delivery. Funding should not be categorical; that is it should not be tied in static fashion to a programme or a category of programmes. Rather, it should be attached to the service user and should follow that person as needs change or he/she moves on to another part of the system. Categorical funding creates artificial barriers to service accessibility and restricts creativity in the design and implementation of services.

TABLE 3

MAJOR THEMES FROM THE LITERATURE ON "WRAP AROUND" SERVICES

- Building and maintaining normal lifestyles.

- Client-centred services that are flexible and include planning for the long-term.

- Provision of unconditional care.

- Working toward less restrictive settings.

- Flexible funding of services.

- Measurable accountability for service outcomes.

There are strong thematic similarities among these 3 different segments of the literature. However, it must be recognised that they all reflect the perspective of the providers.

What about the **perspective of the service users?** What do the consumers say about what they need and want to become independent in the community? Not surprisingly, the service users emphasize consumer choice and active participation in all aspects of service planning, and they advocate for more user-led programmes (Deegan, 1992, Chamberlain, 1978, Salem et al., 1988). They also advocate services and supports to be delivered in more normal and less restrictive settings, and for those services to be funded with flexible monies that are attached to the consumer, not to programmes (Chamberlain & Rogers, 1990, Rogers & Centifanti, 1988).

TABLE 4

MAJOR THEMES FROM THE LITERATURE ON CONSUMER ADVOCACY

- Normal and stable housing in the community.

- Services in least restrictive settings.

- Job training and employment or other consistent sources of financial support.

- Consumer advocacy and involvement in service planning, both at the individual level and at the system level.

- Self-help programmes and user-led programmes.

- Flexible funding that follows the individual.

This brief review of several diverse segments of the literature, each coming from a different perspective, has shown a considerable degree of consistency in describing what it takes to successfully support people with persistent and long-term mental health needs in the community. This convergence of thinking among providers with a different orientation, and among providers and consumers, is quite powerful and sets a clear path for the emerging community care system in Scotland and elsewhere in the United Kingdom.

Housing and supportive services have a critical role to play in successful community care systems. The perceptions of the service users become quite divergent from those of many service providers when housing and supports are considered. Group homes and other forms of congregate housing programmes are the most prevalent model of community housing in most mental health systems in both the United States and the United Kingdom.

However, a recent study (Tanzman, 1993) provides compelling evidence that such models are not the preference of most service users. Tanzman reviewed 43 difference surveys conducted between 1986 and 1992 which assessed consumer preferences for housing and support services. Most mental health service users prefer to live in their own apartments, flats or houses and NOT in mental health residential programmes or group homes. They prefer to live alone or with a spouse, friend or others with whom THEY CHOOSE to live. Users prefer NOT to live with other mental health service users. Most service users recognise their need for supportive services, but they want the supports to be available wherever they live, not just in or near hospitals or traditional residential programme settings. They want supports that are flexible and available on an as needed basis, rather than a constant basis. They want to be able to reach staff who can provide support when they need them, but very few service users actually want to live with such staff. In addition to emotional and social supports, they want material supports such as housing subsidies or benefits, income benefits, transport services, etc.

Reasonable housing, that ranks high in consumer satisfaction is a major factor in achieving successful community integration and tenure. Providers and purchasers of community care services should give attention to the importance of successful matches between service users and their residential environments. Such matches must be defined as much by consumer choice and satisfaction as by objective attributes such as bed capacity, staff-to-resident ratios, etc. service systems should be encouraged to go beyond the common solution of providing residential and support services through group homes and other congregate care schemes. The development of innovative, flexible and cost-efficient schemes that are more consistent with consumer preferences and have the added advantage of not requiring substantial capital investment are advocated. Supported living programmes are one example of such a scheme.

Lifeways Community Care (formerly known as Mentor Community Care) provides individualised residential placements in private homes that are intensively supervised and supported by professional teams for 1400 persons with serious levels of disability in the United States and in the United Kingdom; such schemes can create more opportunity and choice for service users.

REFERENCES

Anthony, W. (1979). The principles of psychiatric rehabilitation. Baltimore: University Park Press.

Anthony, W., Cohen, M., & Farkas, M. (1990). Psychiatric rehabilitation. Boston: Centre for Psychiatric Rehabilitation at Boston University.

Blanch, A., Carling, P., & Ridgeway, P. (1988). Normal housing with specialized support: A psychiatric rehabilitation approach to living in the community. Rehabilitation Psychology, 32(4), 47-55.

Brown, M. A., & Wheeler, T. (1990). Supported housing for the most disabled: Suggestions for providers. Psychosocial Rehabilitation Journal, 13(4), 59-68.

Burchard, J. D., & Clark, R. T., (1990). The role of individualised care in a service delivery system for children and adolescents with severely maladjusted behaviour. The Journal of Mental Health Administration, 17, 48-60.

Campenelli, P.C., Sacks, J. Y., Heckart, K., Ades, Y. J., Frecknall, P., & Yee, P. (1992). Integrating psychiatric rehabilitation within a community residence framework. Psychosocial Rehabilitation Journal, 16(1), 135-153.

Carling, P. (1990). Supported housing: An evaluation agenda. Psychosocial Rehabilitation Journal, 13(4), 95-104.

Carling, P., Randolph, F., Blanch, A., & Ridgeway, P. (1987). Rehabilitation research review: Housing and community integration for people with psychiatric disabilities (National Rehabilitation Information Center Review). Washington, DC: Data Institute.

Chamberlin, J. (1978). On our own: Patient controlled alternatives to the mental health system. New York: McGraw-Hill.

Chamberlin, J., & Rogers, J. A. (1990). Planning a community-based mental health system: Perspectives of service recipients. American Psychologist, 45(11), 1241-1244.

Cohen, M. R. (1989). Integrating psychiatric rehabilitation into mental health systems. In M. D. Farkas and W. A. Anthony (Eds.), Psychiatric rehabilitation programs: Putting theory into practice. Baltimore: Johns Hopkins University press (pp. 162-170, 188-191).

Deegan, P. E. (1992). The independent living movement and people with psychiatric disabilities: Taking back control over our own lives. Psychosocial Rehabilitation Journal, 15(3), 3-19.

Livingston, J. A., Srebnik, D., King, D. A., & Gordon, L. (1992). Approaches to providing housing and flexible supports for people with psychiatric disabilities. Psychosocial Rehabilitation Journal, 16(1), 27-43.

Rogers, J. A., & Centifanti, J. B., (1988). Madness, myths and reality: response to Roberta Rose. Schizophrenia Bulletin, 14, 7-15.

Salem, D. A., Seidman, E., & Rappaport, J. (1988). Community treatment of the mentally ill: The promise of mutual-help organizations. Social Work, 33, 403-408.

Tanzman, B., (1993). An overview of surveys of mental health consumers' preferences for housing and support services. Hospital and Community Psychiatry, 44(5), 450-455.

Van Den Berg, J. E., (1993). Integration of individualised mental health services into the system of care for children and adolescents. Administration and Policy in Mental Health, 20(4), 247-257.

SERVICES FOR THE ELDERLY

DONALD LYONS

In many ways, old age psychiatry is well ahead of general adult psychiatry in the field of community care. This has been achieved, not through increased resources being provided to the mental health services, but by using existing personnel to integrate with other agencies involved in the care of the elderly mentally ill. The South Glasgow services have "networked out" and liaised with social work, private, church and voluntary agencies to deliver quality mental health care.

The major impetus for change has been geographical. The South East Glasgow Sector is served by a remote mental hospital (Leverndale) with poor transport links. While the inpatient assessment unit is still based at Leverndale Hospital, a day hospital adjacent to the catchment area has been developed and this site is also used for outpatient clinics. Community nursing services operate from this base and from a local health centre and there has been a six-fold increase in the number of community nurses in the last 4 years. More recently, all continuing care beds for dementia sufferers have been transferred from Leverndale Hospital to a partnership development with a private company, offering 90 continuing care places in the heart of the catchment area. There is a projected second partnership development in another part of South Glasgow. This has led to the closure of geographically and physically unsuitable accommodation at Leverndale Hospital.

Networking out has taken the form of the following additional services provided by other agencies. **Williamwood House** is a 30 place Church of Scotland Home for the confused elderly was opened in 1982 and the Leverndale consultants are involved in screening referrals and in liaison work. **Dixon Community** is largely a voluntary agency providing day care and home support for the elderly in the Govanhill area of Glasgow. One of the Leverndale consultants is vice-chairman of the Dickson Halls Committee and there is close working between the agencies. **Blairtum Elderly Resource Centre** opened in 1990, it is a social work day care and respite care centre for confused elderly and has had regular psychiatry input from the outset and has been the basis for joint assessment work. **Walker House Dementia Unit** is a 10 based bedded residential unit for dementia sufferers and was recently altered to provide accommodation resembling a 1940's tenement and has proved to be a great success with its clients and with the local community. There is regular psychiatric input and a direct access for the mental health service to some places there. **"Roving Clinic"** is a roving psychiatric clinic established in recognition of the psychiatric morbidity in residential homes; it is taken around all local authority residential care homes with an opportunity for care staff to refer directly for psychiatric advice, albeit with the consent of the patients own general practitioner (GP).

The effect of these service developments has been to increase the number of elderly people with psychiatric morbidity seen by the service and to enable a larger number to be treated without hospital admission. The service has been expanded further by an enhanced multi- disciplinary community team for the locality and the prospects for the future are exciting.

TABLE 1

THE CHANGING FACE OF OLD AGE PSYCHIATRY
IN GLASGOW (SOUTH EAST)

	1989	1994
ACUTE BEDS	60	60
CONTINUING CARE BEDS	135	15
PARTNERSHIP BEDS	0	75
COMMUNITY STAFF	1	15
OUT PATIENT CLINICS	1	5
DAY HOSPITAL (places per week)	60	84

SERVICES FOR THE ELDERLY

CHRISTINE KIRK

Over the last 8 years the strategy for elderly mentally ill people and their carers in York has involved a move from a hospital based service to a community based service. Two psychiatric hospitals have been or are scheduled for closure, (Naburn Hospital closed in 1987 and Clifton Hospital will close in 1994). A network of Community Units for the Elderly (CUEs) providing residential care (continuing care and flexible respite care), day care, domiciliary outreach work, a staff base for community multidisciplinary team members, and a resource centre are being established each to service an elderly catchment population of about 5,000. Four such units have been established, one is being built at the moment and another is planned to open in 1994 in a joint enterprise with social services in a local authority residential home. Another CUE will be built and opened in 1995 and this will complete the strategy.

Assessment facilities are available for elderly people at Bootham Park Hospital with separate facilities for organically and functionally ill people and there is a 20 bedded joint geriatric/psychogeriatric assessment unit with its own dedicated multidisciplinary team in York District Hospital (adjacent to Bootham Park Hospital). As the strategy has continued and the sector mental health teams have established themselves and worked closely with the existing community networks, more and more of the assessment of elderly people has occurred in their own homes and in day care settings resulting in proportionately fewer people being admitted to hospital for assessment. In this way their ongoing management has remained in the community.

In building up the comprehensive range of services there has been close planning with York social services department, voluntary agencies, primary care and carers of existing patients.

An example of the close working with social services is the special home care project with home care assistants being managed by social services but day to day work with patients being co-ordinated with community psychiatric nurses (CPNs) and staff from the CUEs. An evening support service is also being piloted, building on the strength of the home care assistants/CUE staff links. Links with primary care, in particular with general practitioners are fostered by the general practitioners remaining involved with the patients in the CUEs whether they are day visitors or residents.

Many lessons have been learned in the transition in York from traditional hospital based care to the community based services. A detailed evaluation was carried out through support from Research and Development for Psychiatry (RDP) with funding from the Gatsby Charitable Foundation and York Health Authority [Community Units for the Elderly in York Health District: An Evaluation of the first Cue, Acomb Gables - Ann H Pattie and Sallie Moxon - Evaluation & Research Support Unit, Psychology Services, Clifton Hospital, York YO3 6RD (1991)]. Further evaluative work has been carried out by the Evaluation & Research Support Unit and details are available from Sallie Moxon there. The following is a quote from the summary of the report of the evaluation of the first CUE.

"The findings of the evaluation, together with the views of senior staff, are considered to point to appropriateness and success of the strategy for the mental health services for the Elderly. The CUES are seen as offering a quality of service liked by carers, relatives and patients. The staff enjoy working in the service and feel the facilities offered are better for its users and wider community. Since it appears to be no more expensive than traditional services and the waiting lists are certainly no longer, it is considered that the strategy should continue, with services developed along the lines planned, but retaining flexibility to meet changing patterns of need, finance or policies".

Further details of the work contained in this brief summary can be obtained from Dr. Christine Kirk, Consultant Psychiatrist for the Elderly, Bootham Park Hospital, York, YO3 7BY, Tel No: 0904 454071.

REFERENCE

Thompson A & Mathias P. Balilliere Tindall. "Developing a Supportive Service: A Case Example", page 504. Lyttle's Mental Health & Disorder, 2nd Edition, 1994.

CHILD AND ADOLESCENT SERVICES - COMMISSIONING CHILD AND ADOLESCENT MENTAL HEALTH SERVICES

RICHARD WILLIAMS and MICHAEL FARRAR

INTRODUCTION

This chapter, based on a workshop delivered at the Scottish Conference on Mental Health, outlines the current status of child and adolescent mental health services in Britain and endeavours to suggest matters which should receive priority in, first sustaining and second developing, rationally based child and adolescent mental health services.

It is proposed that child and adolescent health services:

- Have been and remain at risk

  This is thought to be the case not least as a consequence of:

  - lack of understanding of the nature and extent of disorder in young people and of the capacities and achievements of services

  - less than appropriate clarity on, and agreement about, the aims, intentions, models, structure and organisational patterns of services

  - Have arrived in this circumstance as a result of the unintended interaction of a variety of factors

  - Would be aided in gaining a more secure place in the spectrum of services through the application of a commissioning process

Such a process could aid services to:

- achieve greater clarity of purpose

- become more equitably distributed

- demonstrate their potential quality and effectiveness

ISSUES WHICH HAVE LED TO THE CURRENT CIRCUMSTANCES -

The Nature and Origin of Present Problems

Over a significant period of time, there has, apparently, been a growing sense of unease about the strategies for, roles assigned to, and the spread of provision of child and adolescent mental health services. These concerns have been voiced by the managers of local authority and health services and by professional staff. Judging by the number of requests for advice received by the NHS Health Advisory Service from Regional Health Authorities (RHAs), Health Authorities (HAs), NHS Trusts and others, these concerns continue and are growing. Recently, the current position, as described based by responses to self report questionnaires sent to all appropriate health and local authority purchasers and providers in England, has been reviewed comprehensively by Kurtz and Wolkind.

Historically, the circumstances and processes which appear to have contributed to this uncertain situation include (Williams, 1992):

- Low levels of accurate awareness of the growing prevalence and the nature of mental disorder in young people

  Awareness of the reality of the extent and short and long-term impacts of mental health problems (including more serious disorders) is only gradually becoming recognised by those with the strategic ability to influence service provision, despite the existence of a growing and substantial body of information over many years.

- Perceived problems in describing and measuring the work of child and adolescent mental health services

  In a similar way, the broad nature and the styles of approach to understanding and interventions appropriate for young people with mental health problems have not leant themselves to simple description and measurement. This problem has been compounded by differences in terminology used by, and the styles of approach of, the differing agencies. Nonetheless, the literature on the effectiveness of a variety of interventions has grown.

- Stigma

  Though children with problems tend generally to be viewed more benignly when compared to adults, stigma relating to mental health problems affecting children and their families continues to exist.

- The inherited historical patchy provision of a diverse range of services

  Though the last 70 years have seen rapid advances in the capacity and provision of child and adolescent mental health services, the greater economic austerity of the mid-seventies caught them in a metaphorical frost at a time when they were at a sensitive point in development. Nonetheless, some advances, including the notable expansion of the academic base, have continued.

- The impact of positive professional developments

  The training and calibre of individuals entering the professions which work with troubled children have improved rapidly. However, in parallel with greater economic austerity following the mid-seventies, services were reaching their own adolescence and a number of the professions, which had previously worked together closely, seemed to need to exercise their own autonomy. This put pressure on the cohesiveness of multidisciplinary teams.

- The impact of service reorganisation

  Whilst many would agree that the introduction of general management in the NHS in 1992 has resulted in clearer systems for service leadership and management, this process greatly accelerated a process of service reform which can be traced to the present. There have been changes in the size, nature and functioning of the responsible health and local authority authorities. As this chapter is written, these changes are still bedding-in. All of this has appeared to have two significant impacts on mental health services for children and adolescents. First, the initially smaller, and now re-enlarging sizes of health authorities, coupled with the greater distance between them as purchasers and the Trusts providing services, have made the specification and achievement of comprehensive mental health services for children more difficult. Second, the inevitable pre-occupation of the health and local authorities with managing these changes has resulted in mental health services for children receiving less attention than their maintenance and development have appeared to need.

- The results of pressures on local authorities

  Throughout the last 25 years, local authorities have been faced with responding to increasing public concern about the care of children. Rapidly increased awareness of the physical, sexual and emotional abuse of minors has been a major matter which has increased and changed the pressures on service at a time when local authorities have had to consider how they should respond to their responsibilities for an enlarging number of older people. Legislation, such as the Education Act 1981, the Children Act 1989 and the NHS and Community Care Act 1990 have brought further changes to the profile of demand on local authorities and the professional staff they employ. The result has been a paradoxical increase in the strain on multidisciplinary teams in the specialist child and adolescent mental health services and, in a significant number of cases, local authority dis-investment in jointly provided services.

COMMISSIONING HEALTH SERVICES

The Seven Stepping Stones

`Purchasers have a responsibility to force the pace of change. Their goal is to improve health and health services, and to change inappropriate ways of delivering clinical care and preventing illness. To achieve this end they need to work for local people.' (NHS Management Executive (NHSME, 1993). The new framework of the NHS and social services requires the shared commitment of both providers and commissioners. The commissioners include health authorities (HAs), family health service authorities (FHSAs), general practitioner fundholders (GPFHs) and local authority social services (SSDs) and education departments (LEAs). The providers include NHS Trusts, the remaining HA directly managed units (DMUs), SSDs, schools (now locally managed), voluntary and non-statutory sector organisations and private sector agencies.

Key issues for commissioners are set out in Table 1 below. These items come from Purchasing for Health - A framework for Action (NHSME, 1993) and are matters which commissioners have been asked to consider for all health services. So, they apply equally to mental health services for young people, though the complexity of organisation and breadth of community orientated services for them impose particular interpretations of each.

Table 1

The Seven `stepping stones' for effective purchasing

- Strategy
- Effective Contracts
- Knowledge-Base
- Responsiveness to Local People
- Mature Relationships with Providers
- Local Alliances
- Organisational Capacity

The Commissioning Process

At this point it is appropriate to distinguish between the meanings of the terms `commissioning' and `purchasing'. Purchasing for Health uses the word `purchasing'. In day-to-day transactions, there is a tendency to use the terms interchangeably. However, in this section of this chapter `commissioning', is taken to refer to a strategically driven process which endeavours to provide effective services of types and in ways which recognise the needs and opinions of an identified population for which they are intended. `Purchasing' is taken to describe a series of technical procedures whereby purchasers relate to providers in securing and monitoring the services they require. Commissioning thus encompasses purchasing but it also implies a greater range of tasks as it involves attempts to monitor, define and manage the market.

It is also appropriate to recognise the differences of approach which are being taken generally by local and health authorities. The former, with conspicuous responsibilities for care management, tend to purchase packages of care for individuals whilst health authorities buy sectors of care for populations. One result of this difference is that assessment of individuals is, at least in part, a purchasing role in the case of local authorities, whilst it lies, almost entirely, within the provider province in the NHS. Indeed HAs are being urged to move away from the extra-contractual referral of individual or small numbers of cases (with HAs employing a variety of techniques including consortium and lead purchasing or giving established ECR budgets to providers with the intention of re-distributing financial risk). Not withstanding these differences in approach which must be surmounted in coming to jointly agreed strategies and priorities and in co-ordinating the care of individuals, local authorities and health purchasers are being encouraged towards joint commissioning. Thus, the sequence of commissioning tasks highlighted in Table 2 could apply in general terms of principle to both sectors.

Table 2

Steps in The Commissioning Process

    1.   **Strategy Formation**

    2.   **Determination of Priorities**

        through conducting a

        a.   **Health Needs Assessment**

        and then

        b.   **Setting Appropriate Local Goals**

        which take full account of

        i.   **The Clinical Realities**

        set against

        ii.   **Knowledge of the Health Gain Issues**

        and, vitally, are influenced by

        iii.   **The Views of Users and Carers**

        But, the priorities set for each area must be realistic in recognising the historically inherited pattern of service delivery and the demands posed by decisions to move committed investments and yet not disrupt services unacceptably. Consequently, it is vital that commissioners have accurate knowledge of the services they are already buying, are advised by their providers and are aware of what they can expect of mature services through:

    c.   **Compiling a Resource Inventory/Map**

        and

    d.   **Consideration of the Visions, Aspirations, Advice and Business Plans of their Providers**

The priorities, once determined, can then inform

3.   **The Generation of an Outline Service Specification**

4.   **Consideration of Service Options**

5.   **Planning the Agenda for Change and Implementation of the Strategy**

6.   **Confirmation of the Service Specification**

7.   **Contract Negotiation and Agreement**

8.   **Monitoring and Outcome Evaluation**

This Table also illustrates the intention of distinguishing `commissioning' from `purchasing' and, thereby, illuminates the overall thesis of this chapter. The contention is that application of a robust, yet co-operative and mature approach, to the strategic process of designing child and adolescent mental health services could benefit the care and treatment of children and adolescents who suffer mental health problems. It would also contribute to a co-ordinated approach to improving the short and long-term mental health of families.

A VISION FOR COMPREHENSIVE CHILD AND ADOLESCENT MENTAL HEALTH SERVICES

The overall goal should be that of providing seamless, multi-sectoral mental health services for children, adolescents and their families which are effective, sensitive and appropriate to the needs of the local population and based on achieving the best from partnerships in care.

Based on awareness of the status of current service provision, the following components of child and adolescent mental health services are seen as requiring particular attention:

- Ensuring that there is a comprehensive pattern of local primary and secondary level services with assured access to specialised and residential tertiary level services

- There is a particular need to endeavour to define and identify a primary level of service from the many professional staff of many sectors who contribute through their work with children with mental health problems

- The integration of purchasing strategies and services provided by a range of statutory and non-statutory services

- Integration of community and hospital services

- Definition, specification and contracting for the provision of liaison, consultation and training services

In addition, the following process issues are considered to require particular attention.

- The specification of services needs to be viewed from the client perspective

With respect to children, adolescents and families, this involves:

- Adoption of developmental and life-cycle foci

There is also need for:

- Clear referral guidelines/protocols

Services need to be multi-sectoral as no one statutory agency can establish a comprehensive range of services on its own. However, without continuing discussion and liaison at both commissioning and providing levels, misunderstandings between agencies can, all too easily, arise resulting in uncertainty, confusion and sometimes disagreement about the definition of the client groups, referral pathways and service priorities. This depends on purchaser and provider:

- Partnerships and alliances with and within the full range of child health services

and:

- Partnerships between the local authority SSD and LEA and the mental health services for children

and:

- Partnerships with other services for children (eg the Courts)

A STRATEGIC APPROACH TO THE PROVISION OF CHILD AND ADOLESCENT MENTAL HEALTH SERVICES

Some of the issues identified above as requiring particular consideration in moving towards commissioning comprehensive mental health services for children and adolescents are now presented under the headings derived from the Seven Stepping Stones in Purchasing for Health. The intention is to identify an approach which is compatible with that which the NHS Executive has been presenting to health purchasers in the belief that, well handled locally, such an approach could benefit the development of services in the desired directions.

Strategy

- Joint ownership

  Ideally, the commissioning strategy for each population should be jointly owned by each of the purchasing agencies. Wherever possible, joint commissioning is to be encouraged but, when not, strategies should be jointly agreed and co-ordinated by the purchasing organisations which include HAs and GPFHs and the social services and education departments of the local authorities.

- Long-Termism

  The crucial tasks for commissioners of ensuring comprehensive, integrated services, in which effective and broadly-based community services are developed to work alongside modern specialised hospital facilities of adequate volume and quality, demand that a long term approach to strategy is taken in alliance with crucial service partners.

- Defining and describing mental health problems and definition of the client groups

  A crucial matter in strategy development is that of defining the client groups. This must be agreed between the purchasing agencies in any district, in their harmonisation of strategy, and between purchasers and providers, in order to secure complimentary and well co-ordinated services. Commissioners should ensure that all with the most severe problems and disorders are offered effective services and support. In their strategies, commissioners should agree a profile of provision which balances recognition of the importance of the needs of young people with the most demanding problems with the needs of those with less serious problems.

- Needs assessment and agency needs assessments

  Needs assessment must not only reflect national data but should also be tuned by the addition of locally derived information drawn from the sources available to a wide range of service purchasing and providing partners. The multi-sectoral broad span of services required and the wide range of avenues of presentation of young people and their families demand that liaison, consultation and training offered by the specialised services are seen as important, main-stream aspects of mature provision. Thus the needs of health and non-health agencies for these collaborative aspects of service should be recognised in the strategy and supported by the contracts which run from it.

- Definition/creation of an identifiable primary mental health service

  Much of the concentration of concern about child and adolescent mental health services from within the NHS has been about the adequacy of provision of specialist, secondary and tertiary, levels of care. This has been appropriate but does not represent the full spectrum of what is required. Traditionally, persisting child and adolescent mental health problems and disorders, other than minor ones, have been seen as the province of specialist services. Recently, there has been greater emphasis on the contributions which could be made to a comprehensive pattern of service by primary health care teams (PHCTs). Local authority education and social services departments make significant primary level investments in services which deal directly and indirectly with young people who have a range of mental health problems. They have also made direct contributions, jointly with the NHS, to specialist secondary and tertiary level services, though their contributions to jointly provided and managed services have declined significantly in the last ten years. It is also likely that significant primary level mental health interventions are offered by the NHS through health visitors, GPs etc, but these have not been recognised as contributing to an identified mental health service. It is suggested that this situation has contributed to:

- under-recognition of the contributions made to mental health services for children, adolescents and families made by a variety of professionals including teachers, social workers, GPs and health visitors

- lack of definition and recognition of a strategically planned and tasked primary level mental health service for children and adolescence with consequent:

- reliance on specialist secondary level services

- uncertainty about referral protocol and differing practices relating to access to and client selection by the specialist services

- the difficulties which have sometimes arisen between the staff of specialist in child and adolescent mental health services in agreeing service priorities when faced with demands which are greater than the supply.

It is suggested that identification and better strategic definition of the actual and potential contributions and contributors to a primary level service in each area would move towards resolving some of these problems and achieving services which are more comprehensive overall.

Effective Contracts

In the past, many contracts have been concerned with sustaining a historically defined level of service volume and quality. The development of child and adolescent mental health services requires changes in their structure and functioning and, thus, in investment in them. This requires a thorough knowledge of need in each local population coupled with a working knowledge of information relating to health gain for each client group.

These two matters should be considered together with information on the views of users and carers and the practical clinical realities in determining strategies for the shape, nature and monitoring of contracts.

As for the design of strategy, the specification of services also requires a multi-agency approach. In some cases, collaboration may proceed incrementally from *complementary purchasing,* with full sharing of information, planned changes and developments, through *joint specification,* to *joint purchasing* with resources from health commissioners and local authority departments being deployed through single contracts.

Service specifications should deal with the items considered in the section on strategy. Additionally, and of particular importance in services for children and adolescents, the interfaces between services and consideration of the management of referrals across boundaries set by age are important in ensuring seamless services.

There are a number of other matters to which commissioners might also pay attention in contracting and these include:

- An adequate contract framework for voluntary and non-statutory sector providers

    Voluntary and non-statutory organisations provide a significant volume and range of services for children who are at a substantially increased risk of suffering serious mental health problems and disorders. Therefore, commissioners should find effective contractual mechanisms and frameworks to sustain these important service partners.

- Contract currencies

    Commissioners should recognise that simple contract currencies, such as the Finished Consultant Episode (FCE) do not recognise the breadth of functioning of comprehensive child and adolescent mental health services. On their own, these currencies are likely to be insufficient to address the full range of what is required.

- Involvement of the clinical professions in contracting

    The potential for misunderstanding what good mental health services can and cannot achieve accentuates the importance of the professionals, who deliver services, being involved in contract negotiation. Also the range of professional disciplines appropriately involved in providing mental health services is broad which further emphasises the crucial importance to commissioners of their receiving good professional advice to sit alongside that received from the users of services and their carers.

- Purchasing low volume specialised services

    Some young people with severe mental health problems and illnesses require the provision of very specialised services. In some cases, the numbers of people concerned are relatively low and it would not be reasonable or economic for purchasers to expect each of their providers to offer these services locally. However, each purchaser should ensure that it has contracts with providers for these services. Examples include specialist eating disorder services, inpatient and day services for adolescents and secure forensic services for mentally disordered adolescent offenders. A practical guide on Contracting for Specialised Services was published by the NHSME in 1993. Some of the client groups are very small in number and these situations may require a broader approach to service commissioning on a semi-national or national basis. The NHS Health Advisory Service is able to offer advice on a number of options as to how this task might be handled in the reformed health and welfare services.

Knowledge-Base

The rapid growth in knowledge specifically about mental health matters affecting children and their families should be recognised by commissioners who need to develop a base-line level of knowledge and mechanisms for updating themselves.

Key issues include:

- Identifying the population of concern

- Developing information systems

    These activities should be developed in conjunction with providers. Commissioners should balance their requests for information such that they are enabled to specify and monitor the services they procure without becoming involved in either the management of those services or limiting proper clinical discretion which are the legitimate roles of providers.

A vital function for commissioners is that of:

- Mapping the current provision of services

    It is important that commissioners should have an accurate knowledge of the nature, distribution and capacity of the services which are available. Such a resource inventory will promote the efficient and effective use of current facilities and form an essential baseline for service development. Mapping services for children and adolescents is particularly important as purchasers cannot make assumptions about local provision due to the sporadic nature of their development across the country, variations in style and approach, and the multi-sectoral contributions to care which are required.

Commissioners should set early local objectives for improving their knowledge-base. In addition to accessing the sources considered above, this will involve:

- Developing mechanisms for receiving information from a variety of other local agencies, such as the courts etc.

- Establishing mechanisms for user and carer relationships

- Establishing mechanisms for receiving high quality professional advice

- Undertaking prospective local research.

Responsiveness To Local People

This role includes, but is also more complex than, simply asking local populations to help identify local health priorities. It is important for commissioners to avoid reinforcing stereotypes and the stigma which is associated with mental health problems and disorder.

Commissioners need to sustain and develop skills for engaging with the public through the use of local media, publishing service information, developing new relationships with the Community Health Councils, offering financial support for self-help schemes, and stimulating user-led lobbying groups, amongst other activities.

Of particular importance are:

- User and carer involvement

  Commissioners need mechanisms for involving users and carers and consulting them on the planning, development and improvement of local services and on their purchasing intentions. There are particular challenges to face in involving children and adolescents, though they are by no means insurmountable.

- Setting quality standards for, and the assessment of, local provision

- Identifying lessons from experience and research

- A well structured `stakeholder' dialogue

  Purchasers should keep stakeholders or their representatives fully informed and consulted about priorities and plans. The dialogues with stakeholders can aid:

  - the assessment of what is happening now

  - decisions on priorities for improvement

  - mobilising action to plan for change and development

Purchasers should recognise that certain individuals and groups will take up roles as 'product champions'. In turn, purchasers should become the champions of the consultative process whereby all views are taken into account.

Mature Relationships With Providers

Although relationships with providers are defined through contracting, contracting is a technical function the impact of which is likely to be effected significantly by the more general nature of the relationship between each purchaser and provider.

Mental health services are essentially complex and multi-faceted. So, perhaps more than in any other service arena, successful mental health services for children and adolescents will depend on effective partnerships between purchasers, who should set the strategy, and providers, who should enact it. A positive partnership involves sharing risk at a variety of levels, sharing expertise in improving the mental health status of populations, the effective targeting of resources at those young people with the most severe needs without forgetting the needs of those with less severe problems and the avoidance of unnecessary use of resource to rectify disagreement.

The development of effective partnerships should be led from the Chair of the HA, and SSD and Education Committee and each of the relevant Trusts. These initiatives should be communicated to, and resonate through, all levels of staff in all the organisations involved.

Experience has shown that attention to the quality of purchaser-provider relationships at all levels does much to promote the quality of mental health services generally and the resolution of strategic and resourcing disagreements. However, of particular importance to children and adolescents with more severe mental disorders are:

- The co-ordination of care programmes and care management policies and procedures

- Co-ordination of policies, procedures and practice to ensure:

    - the identification of priority groups

    - agencies work together to secure a unified and coherent approach to care

    - continuity of care

    - each agency discharges its responsibility for accountability.

Local Alliances

Working across agency and disciplinary boundaries is a necessity for commissioners, if they are to improve the mental health of the young people in the populations for which they are responsible. Purchasers should establish a well defined process by which they are to work with others to improve local systems of service delivery.

Organisational Capacity

Achieving the strategic development of mental health service, such that they become more accessible, responsive, comprehensive, modern and better integrated, places a significant burden on both purchasers and providers.

Issues important in developing the organisational capacities of these organisations in responding to the challenges include the attitudes and skills of all concerned. This is particularly the case for commissioners who have had to learn a new set of skills very rapidly. These skills must be tailored to the needs of young people with mental health problems. Negative attitudes to the value and impact of mental health services need to be challenged as should stigma, wherever it occurs. So the beliefs and knowledge of commissioners are important in shaping mental health services.

WHAT IS BEING DONE

In recognition of the current circumstances of child and adolescent mental health services, the NHS Health Advisory Service (HAS) has been asked to conduct a Thematic Review to formulate advice on the Commissioning and Management of Child and Adolescent Mental Health Services. This will examine the issues raised in this chapter and others in greater depth. The work will be based on both theoretical consideration and fieldwork designed to explore the current, but historically derived, position, collate good practice and benchmark possible recommendations.

The Thematic Review will offer advice at national level which will be tuned to local requirements with the intention of aiding purchasing/commissioning authorities in developing their Knowledge-Base and Organisational Capacities.

In parallel, the HAS is undertaking a variety of assignments to advise Ministers, RHAs, DAs and local authorities on their approaches to a variety of matters in the design and evaluation of child and adolescent mental health services.

References and Bibliography

A Unique Window on Change - The Annual Report of the Director of the NHS Health Advisory Service for 1992-93, (1993).
London: HMSO.

Purchasing for Health (1993) NHS Management Executive

Williams, R., (1992). The Need to Manage the Market, is With Health in Mind - Proceedings of a Conference.
London: National Association of Health Authorities and Trusts and Action for Sick Children

CHILD AND ADOLESCENT SERVICES - CHILD AND ADOLESCENT PSYCHIATRIC SERVICES IN SCOTLAND

PETER HOARE

Introduction

The recent NHS reforms have forced a radical reappraisal of health care provision. Child and adolescent psychiatry is a small sub-speciality with wide variation in service development and range of services. Parry-Jones (1990, 1992) has written extensively about the opportunities and also the threats that the reforms pose for the speciality. There are no nationally agreed guidelines about minimum service provision except for the pious plea from clinicians for more and more. Smith & Simpson (1994) have recently argued that child and adolescent psychiatry is particularly vulnerable as it is difficult to audit and also, more importantly, to evaluate the effectiveness of child and adolescent psychiatry.

For all these reasons, it seemed timely to obtain accurate information about child and adolescent psychiatry services in Scotland. Consequently, the Executive Committee of the Child and Adolescent Section of the Scottish Division of the Royal College of Psychiatrists commissioned Drs. Morton and Norton, Consultant Psychiatrists with Dumfries and Forth Valley Health Boards respectively, to undertake a questionnaire survey of all consultant child and adolescent psychiatrists in Scotland. This survey was completed in early 1993. The questionnaire had 4 sections: referral patterns; staffing levels; in-patient and day patient services, and a Strength Weaknesses Opportunities Threats (SWOT) analysis of the individual's own clinical service.

This paper describes the results of this survey and its implications for child and adolescent psychiatric service provision in Scotland. I have also undertaken a further analysis of the results from the survey in order to relate referral patterns to demographic characteristics.

Results

Replies were obtained from 34 of the 40 consultants (85% completion rate). Non-responders consisted of 2 consultants who were off sick and four others whose posts were either occupied by a locum or being re-organised.

Referral Patterns

Table 1 summarises the absolute new referral rate according to child population, consultant staffing and total medical staffing for the 12 principal health boards (equivalent to regions in England and Wales). The results show that there is a two-fold variation in referral with rates ranging from 2.4% to 1.14%. There is an even larger variation in the consultant and total medical staff referral rates, 300 to 125 and 240 to 88 respectively. Table 2 ranks the health boards from highest to lowest on the same 3 referral characteristics. It shows that health board 1, a teaching board, has the highest referral rate but is only 7th when referral rate per medical staff member is calculated. Similarly, health board 10 has the 10th referral rate, but the second and third highest rate per consultant and per medical staff member respectively.

Consultant Staffing

Table 3 compares current consultant medical establishment with the Royal College of Psychiatrists' recommendations (Hill 1990). The College produces 2 figures, an absolute minimum level of consultant staff and a higher, more desirable figure, according to the population, the provision of in-patient services and whether the Board is teaching or non-teaching. The results show that only 3 health boards in Scotland are meeting the minimum requirements with none attaining the higher staffing levels.

The SWOT Analysis of the Clinical Service

The respondents consistently identified 4 strengths to their service; the provision of a good local service, committed and dedicated staff, good multidisciplinary team working, and close links with local community and paediatric services. Table 4 summarises the weaknesses: only 25% rated the staff establishment as acceptable or better; accommodation was unsatisfactory or worse in 44%; 20% were dissatisfied with other resources such as equipment or audio-visual facilities; and only 38% gave at least an acceptable rating for their overall service. Thirty five per cent of consultants had little or no ready access to child clinical psychology services, whilst the survey also showed that there was no child psychotherapy post anywhere in the NHS in Scotland. Not surprisingly, the most consistent demand was for more resources.

In-Patient and Day Patient Resources

Child psychiatry in-patient services were available at 5 sites providing a total of 48 beds for children up to 14 years of age. Two units operated a 7 day service with the remainder run on a 5 day basis. The average length of admission was 6 months. Adolescent in-patient services were present at 6 sites with an even distribution of 5 and 7 day units. Average admission time was four and a half months with a total of 55 beds. The survey revealed that 6 Health Boards had no in-patient psychiatric service for children or adolescents.

Most of the in-patient units also ran day patient programmes with one unit established solely to provide a day patient programme.

Discussion

The results of this small survey highlight the wide variation in clinical demand and service provision for child and adolescent psychiatry in Scotland. The striking two-fold difference in referral rate has important implications for service provision locally and nationally. Several factors may be responsible for this variation- inaccurate information, child population differences, age range of the service, teaching versus non-teaching boards, range of services provided, (particularly the availability of in-patient and day patient resources), other local services for disturbed children, and socio-economic factors.

It is unlikely that inaccurate data on referral rates is important as local and national attendance figures have been recorded on a national basis for a long time. Similarly, the percentage of the child population shows little variation between health boards with a range of 3% from 20-23% and most health boards around 21-22%. The age range of the service may be important, particularly with adolescent services. Referral rates may vary considerably depending upon whether the child and adolescent services cease at 16 years of age or continue through to 18 years or older. If the latter is provided by child and adolescent services, assessment of the older adolescent following a self harm episode may have a significant impact on referral patterns. Similar arguments apply to a small number of children or adolescents admitted to in-patient care as a source of variation. Anecdotal evidence suggests that waiting times, not considered in the survey, have an important influence on the utilisation of child and adolescent services. Another crucial, but difficult to quantify factor, is the availability and range of services provided by social services and education. Hoare (1993) discusses the interaction between health, social services and education in service provision for disturbed children and adolescents.

Finally, substantial research, reviewed by Garmezy & Masten (1994) has shown that disturbed children and adolescents are likely to suffer from considerable socio-economic disadvantage. There is a wide variation both between and within health boards with regard to this factor. Unfortunately, the resources of the survey did not permit an adequate assessment of the relevance of this factor.

The consultants' views on staff establishment and resources are perhaps not new or unexpected. Nevertheless, the scarcity of the clinical psychology service, the absence of child psychotherapy posts and the low level of consultant establishment must be dispiriting for the staff in the service. Senior staff were also pessimistic about the likelihood of improvement particularly when competing with general psychiatry and acute medical specialities for scarce resources.

The wide variation in the provision of day and in-patient services has been known for some time, and this survey confirms this situation. The next and more difficult stage is to give a satisfactory explanation for this finding.

Conclusions

This paper has discussed the provision of child and adolescent psychiatric services in Scotland. It has highlighted the sparse data on which the service is purchased and provided a situation that will need to change as the NHS reforms become firmly established. A positive outcome from this situation is that consultant child and adolescent psychiatrists have banded together to conduct a national audit of out-patient services in Scotland. This project has recently obtained funding from the Clinical Resource and Audit Group (CRAG) of the Scottish Home and Health Department. Hopefully, the results should be available for the next meeting about mental health services in Scotland.

REFERENCES

Garmezy N, Masten A 1994 Chronic Adversities In: Rutter M, Hersov L, Taylor E (eds.) Child and Adolescent Psychiatry: Modern Approaches. Oxford: Blackwell Scientific Publications.

Hill, P 1990 Manpower: Regional and National Issues. In: Hendriks JH, Black M (eds.) Child Psychiatry in the Nineties, pp.98-99, London: Royal College of Psychiatrists

Hoare, P 1993 Essential Child Psychiatry Edinburgh: Churchill Livingstone

Parry-Jones, WLI 1990 Economic Appraisal of Child and Adolescent Psychiatry In: Hendriks J H, Black M (eds.) Child Psychiatry in the Nineties, pp.71-73, London: Royal College of Psychiatrists

Parry-Jones WLI 1992 Management in the Health Service in relation to children and the provision of child psychiatric service Association of Child Psychiatry and Psychology Newsletter, 14, 3-10

Smith J, Simpson J 1994 Locally determined performance pay: better levers for improving performance in a health service with disparate values British Medical Journal 309, 493-494.

TABLE 1

REFERRAL PATTERNS

Health Board	Referral Rate/ Population %	Referral Rate/ Consultant	Referral Rate/ Total Medical Staff
1	2.40	268	118
2	2.29	240	240
3	2.06	300	225
4	2.03	125	88
5	1.73	200	150
6	1.66	193	116
7	1.64	150	116
8	1.58	177	101
9	1.46	225	112
10	1.45	275	220
11	1.38	160	162
12	1.14	213	158

TABLE 2

REFERRAL PATTERNS: RANKINGS FROM HIGHEST TO LOWEST

Health Board	Referral Rate/ Population	Referral Rate/ Consultant	Referral Rate/ Total Medical Staff
1	1	3	7
2	2	4	1
3	3	1	2
4	4	12	12
5	5	7	6
6	6	8	9
7	7	11	7
8	8	9	11
9	9	5	10
10	10	2	3
11	11	10	4
12	12	6	5

TABLE 3

CONSULTANT STAFFING

Health Board	Consultants	College Recommendations	
		Irreducible Minimum	Realistically Desirable
1	2.0	3.7	6.0
2	3.0	4.3	6.6
3	0.8	1.0	1.5
4	2.4	2.4	3.6
5	3.0	3.5	5.6
6	3.0	3.0	4.0
7	4.8	7.3	10.7
8	6.0	14.7	22.0
9	2.0	2.0	3.0
10	3.0	5.6	7.5
11	6.7	11.4	18.0
12	3.5	6.4	9.6

TABLE 4

SERVICE ASSESSMENT (WEAKNESSES)

Aspect of Service	Seriously inadequate	Unsatisfactory	Acceptable	Good/Above Average	Excellent
Staff	16	10	4	3	1
Accommodation	4	11	6	9	4
Other Resources	6	3	10	12	3
Rating of Service	9	12	11	2	0

SUBSTANCE ABUSE SERVICES - DRUG MISUSE

J. GREENWOOD

The subject of drug misuse presents a diversity of problems, not only with respect to the strategies which can be employed in dealing with this problem, but also the population involved and the numerous consequences of abuse. In this respect it is very clear that the subject of HIV infection represents an enormous risk to the physical health of misusers.

The strategies for dealing with drug misuse range from in-patient or out-patient care and a rehabilitation service to punishment and the criminal justice system. In practice an enormous emphasis has been placed upon the risk of HIV infection and therefore strong attempts have been made to stop the injecting of drugs. This has had a major effect on the evolution of the service in Edinburgh.

Drugs of misuse can be divided into 2 groups. Firstly, there are the drugs of dependence and these can be approximately divided into tranquillisers and painkillers. Secondly, there are recreational drugs. There is evidence from studies in Manchester that up to 70% of school children may be offered drugs, whilst between 30 and 50% take them, over time. The pattern of use develops from that of experimentation to dependence and the interval between initiation of drug abuse and presentation to the services varies from between 8 to 10 years. Bearing this in mind there are 3 potential focuses for intervention. **Firstly** to stop new recruits. **Secondly,** focus interventions upon those who need intervention, but do not want it. **Thirdly,** focus intervention on those who both need and want it.

Within Lothian Health Board the strategy has been one of harm reduction with 3 main focuses. **Firstly,** provision of exchange facilities, so that less hazardous equipment can be supplied for those injecting, **secondly,** the use of substitute prescribing, **thirdly,** the use of Health Education particularly in a preventative role.

With respect to prescribing this can be viewed both with respect to harm reduction and as a means of developing a therapeutic relationship. The benefits of prescribing Methadone include the following; the conversion from injecting drugs to the use of oral substitutes, the reduction of crime associated with prescribed supply, a general stabilisation in lifestyle, and regular contact with the service. Using prescribing to gain patient contact a therapeutic relationship can be formed leading ultimately to changes in lifestyle and abstinence from drug abuse.

Shared Care

In Lothian this approach to treatment of drug misuse has been used by the Drug Service in liaison with General Practitioners[1,2]. The model of shared care involves community psychiatric nurses and medical specialists who liaise with the general practitioner (GP). In addition there is a primary care facilitator available to train GPs with respect to HIV infection and drug abuse. Referrals to the service come from General Practitioners and after the initial meeting with the community psychiatric nurse (CPN), a management meeting takes place involving the doctor, nurse and user. At that time a plan is agreed and the roles of different professionals made clear. The general practitioner prescribes Methadone and takes physical care of the patient, whilst it is the role of the CPN to maintain regular contact and to initiate counselling. There is a clear understanding that should this regular contact be discontinued, then there will be no further prescribing. Setting up this system involved prolonged discussions between the team and general practitioner.

With this system in place between 1988 and 1992, 2,094 people were referred. In the first year there were 138 referrals, whilst at present there are 800 referrals per year. It is estimated that over that time two thirds of the drug users in Lothian have been referred. Approximately 50% of clients each year continue to be in contact with the service for a subsequent year but given this accumulative load, once stabilised, more clients are now discharged back to their general practitioner (G.P.). Seventy per cent of Lothian GPs prescribe for around 1200 drug users[3], with the Community Drug Problem Service (CDPS) prescribing for 80 of the more difficult cases.

Edinburgh versus Glasgow

There are differences in drug abuse between the cities of Edinburgh and Glasgow (Table). In Edinburgh, the main painkillers used are Dihydrocodeine and Methadone, whilst in Glasgow the main drugs used are Temgesic, Heroin and Diconal. With respect to the tranquilliser group of drugs, in Edinburgh Temazepam is more likely to be used orally, whilst in Glasgow it is more often used by the intravenous route. There is research evidence[4] that attempts to reduce the injecting of drugs in Edinburgh has been more successful in comparison with Glasgow.

In addition to research, the police in Edinburgh have acknowledged a reduction in crime figures with this change in the injecting pattern. Heroin is no longer the major problem that it was previously because of medical services controlling the principal drugs used.

The findings raise a number of important issues. Would the changes in Edinburgh's drug use since the initiation of the policy of shared care have happened anyway? How long can general practitioners sustain this level of input? Should the policy of prescribing Methadone to drug users continue, with the implication of higher numbers of the population receiving this substance? Can this service encourage users to move on to abstinence from drugs? Will there be a new problem created by pharmaceutical dependence?

Discussion

Dr Grant acknowledged the conflict in Glasgow with respect to prescribing Methadone and whilst at present the psychiatric services have agreed by consensus not to prescribe Methadone, at present, in the city one or two GPs are now doing so.

The first question asked referred to the effectiveness of residential rehabilitation facilities and the discussion proceeded thus: the traditional model of removing patients from the area where drugs are available to them appears to be less useful in a contemporary society than it may previously have been. At present there is a preference for dealing with the issue of drug use in the community and a focus placed upon moderating the lifestyle of users. This is much more pertinent and difficult than to withdraw from drugs in an in-patient environment.

The important feature of substitute prescribing is that this allows the service to gain contact with drug users and thereby enables counselling which is the mainstay of treatment. The focus of such an approach is to attempt to improve relationships and move towards a change in lifestyle including issues such as training and remaining outwith the Prison Service. It seems clear that the lives of many drug users is very disturbed prior to treatment interventions. Attention is drawn to the fact that financial savings from the decreased use of the Prison Service are never seen within the National Health Service. None-the-less this sort of approach has many health gains to the affected communities.

The second issue raised was that the focus upon intravenous injectors takes away resources from non-injectors (acknowledging that previous work has reduced the number of injectors). It was acknowledged that certainly in Edinburgh the role of HIV infection has been a major incentive in the development of this service, but that at present in Glasgow there are also fatalities associated with drug injection related to the substances used. The issue of HIV infection has provided funding for the drug abuse service in the past, but at present, in Edinburgh, the experience is that most people being seen in the drug service now have never injected drugs. As a group, drug users are "unpopular" and this has traditionally led to few resources being available to help them until HIV infection became an issue.

A related issue was that of the difficulty experienced in encouraging General Practitioners to be actively involved in the treatment of drug abusers. In this respect the importance of a primary care facilitator was emphasised, as well as the work of the CDPS team which is now sectorized to enhance community and GP links.

Overall, Dr Greenwood suggested that given the present problems associated with drug use in 1993, the best approach was to offer counselling and the prescription of Methadone, given that the client group involved are young, chaotic, immature, disadvantaged, unemployed and often have a sense of hopelessness. The discussion included consideration of community problems and possible solutions, eg the use of "dry cafes", in Shetland. However, it was acknowledged that there has to be some prioritisation of medical activity which can be focused at several levels, which including that of prevention, providing a clinical service and the political lobbying.

The third focus of discussion related to the relationship between drug abuse and the Criminal Justice System. In Edinburgh the Procurator Fiscal Group invite Dr Greenwood to speak annually at their meeting. This is to facilitate a balance in dealing with drug users by punishment and enforcement of the law, whilst at the same time limiting the damage caused by drug use. This raised the issue of legislation regarding risk taking behaviour in general society. However, within the drug service, the view is taken that legal status should not influence the treatment being offered. Whilst there is doubtless an issue relating to prejudice against drug users and the drug user being described as "the witch of the 20th century", there is also a historical move away from the view that users should "go away and come back when you want to stop", and that the view and strategy of harm reduction may well have been galvanised by the effect of HIV infection.

Ethics

The debate was ended by brief mention of the importance of the ethical issues involved in providing a service for intervention which meets the needs of the service user. The prescription of drugs has played its part in the development of dependence and discussion of the iatrogenic problems could include that the prescription of Methoadone.

REFERENCES

1.   Greenwood, J. 1990. Creating a new drug service in Edinburgh. Bri. Med. J. 300. 587-587.

2.   Greenwood, J. 1992. Persuading general practitioners to prescribe good husbandry or a recipe for chaos. Br. Journal of Addiction. 87. 567-575.

3.   Bury, J. 1994. HIV infection and drug misuse in Cohen General Practice. Report on Epidemiological questionnaire 1993. Dr. J. Bury. Lothian Health.

4.   Haw, S. 1993. Pharmaceutical drugs and illicit drug use in Lothian Region. Centre for HIV/Aids and Drug Studies Edinburgh.

PATTERN OF DRUG USE IN EDINBURGH 1992
(N=121)

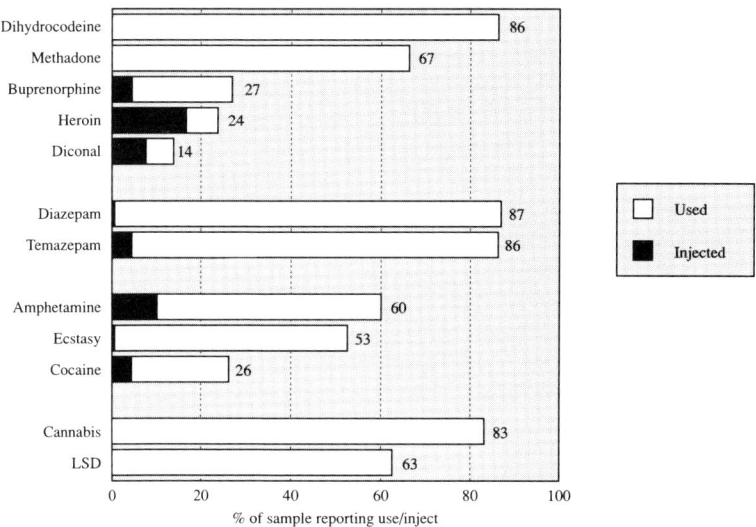

PATTERN OF DRUG USE IN GLASGOW 1991
(N=535)

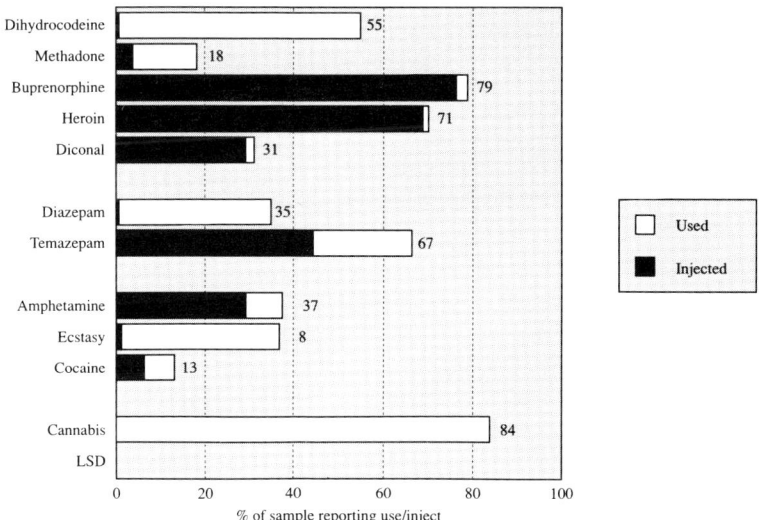

* no data available

SUBSTANCE ABUSE SERVICES - ALCOHOL MISUSE

B. RITSON

Introduction

Alcohol is a our most popular drug. If one considers the whole population who expose themselves to alcohol, then within that group there will be a number whose alcohol intake is hazardous to their health and a smaller number who suffer from alcohol dependence and/or alcohol related problems. The focus of the Alcohol Problems Clinic in Edinburgh is on providing a comprehensive out-patient assessment (see diagram). Subsequently most patients are treated as out-patients, detoxification being conducted at home. There is also a day-patient programme and, for a minority of patients, an in-patient detoxification and treatment programme which makes extensive use of group techniques.

Level of Recognition

Recognition of alcohol associated difficulties may be divided into four levels. The first and most informal is friends and colleagues who may recognise that a problem with alcohol is arising. It is at this level that health promotion in a general sense is most likely to be useful. At the next level there are employers, social welfare agencies, and even bar tenders who encounter the consequences of alcohol problems and may be well placed to offer advice. Alcohol-in-employment policies have been a particularly valuable development. At a third level, generic professional services become involved with individuals who have alcohol problems, most notably general practitioners, accident and emergency staff, police and social work agencies. At the fourth level of response come those whose professional activities are specifically identified with helping this group, such as specialised treatment units, councils on alcohol and Alcoholics Anonymous (AA).

It must always be recognised that the level of alcohol related problems in a community will be influenced by availability and prevailing price and control policies. Preventative action also needs to focus in these areas.

Intervention Levels

Patients drinking in a harmful way may often respond to interventions from primary health care. People with alcohol related problems consult their general practitioners (GPs) more frequently than other similar groups, and focused advice given in this setting is beneficial. Similar observations can be made concerning general hospitals and casualty departments. The extent to which GPs are willing to participate in identifying and managing alcohol problems is debatable. It is clear that support and training would be necessary if this were to become a routine procedure (see DRAMS Scheme).

An unknown proportion of individuals with alcohol problems do not respond to focused advice, often because of the existence of underlying psychological, social or interpersonal problems. In these circumstances further specialist help may be needed. It is in this area that specialist counselling services are most helpful, although their efficacy requires to be evaluated.

Finally there are those patients who have developed advanced alcohol problems, usually with evidence of physical and psychological dependence. In a minority of cases this will be associated with severe social problems such as loss of relationships and homelessness. A further minority will have developed alcohol related physical illnesses including cognitive impairment.

The specialist services themselves include agencies such as the Councils on Alcohol, AA and hospital based services. In recent times there has been interest in community alcohol teams and in this respect there are some parallels between drug and alcohol services eg the parallel between primary care facilitator in the drug services and community nurses working with GPs. (See substance abuse section).

Treatment

There are 5 stages of response to treatment: recognition, motivation, detoxification, active treatment and relapse prevention.

Detoxification from alcohol can be undertaken at home (domiciliary detoxification involving liaison between community nurses and GPs); as an out-patient; day-patient or in-patient.

In line with this variety of settings for alcohol detoxification there is also need for a broad base of treatment options given the many different manifestations of alcohol problems.

The co-ordination and monitoring of services requires further development; the difficulty of identifying the consumer group in order to match its needs to the resources available remains.

Discussion

At present 400 new patients per year are referred to the service in Edinburgh by GPs. The vast majority are seen and treated as out-patients, though some people may need prolonged support. A smaller number enter the day programme. The use of an in-patient detoxification facility is very much limited to the minority. A three week in-patient programme is run in parallel with detoxification to examine the problems associated with alcohol abuse and alternative coping strategies which may be employed. Patients treated in the general psychiatric wards often report feeling misplaced.

"User" Perspective

The view was expressed that the problem of dependence upon prescribed drugs had been

MANAGING ALCOHOL PROBLEMS IN LOTHIAN

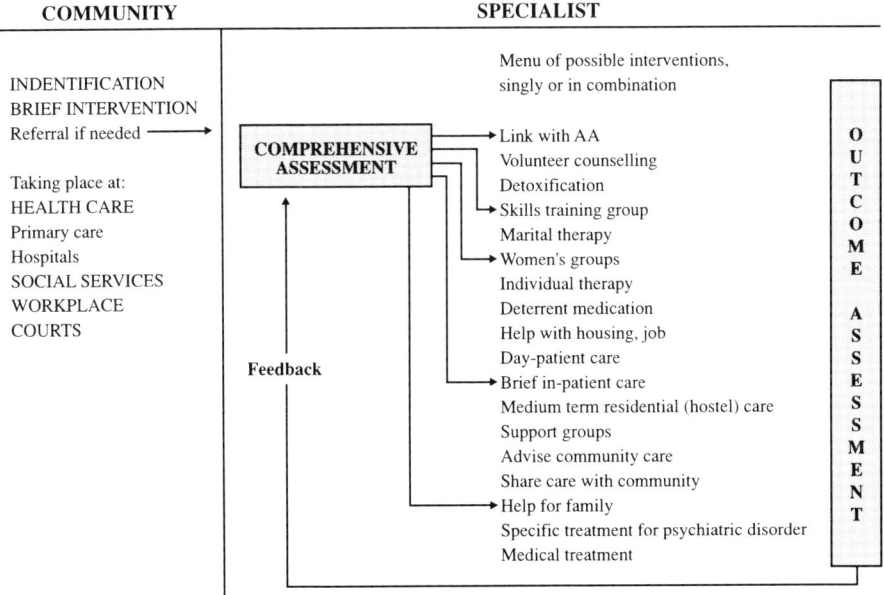

COMMUNITY

INDENTIFICATION
BRIEF INTERVENTION
Referral if needed ⟶

Taking place at:
HEALTH CARE
Primary care
Hospitals
SOCIAL SERVICES
WORKPLACE
COURTS

COMPREHENSIVE ASSESSMENT

Feedback

SPECIALIST

Menu of possible interventions, singly or in combination

Link with AA
Volunteer counselling
Detoxification
Skills training group
Marital therapy
Women's groups
Individual therapy
Deterrent medication
Help with housing, job
Day-patient care
Brief in-patient care
Medium term residential (hostel) care
Support groups
Advise community care
Share care with community
Help for family
Specific treatment for psychiatric disorder
Medical treatment

OUTCOME ASSESSMENT

relatively unrepresented during discussion. There appears to be particular difficulties with the mixed problem of alcohol and Benzadiazepine dependence and it is unclear whether drug and alcohol dependence should be treated together. An issue which may be important in this is how to obtain a representative group of service users to give their view about how they would like interventions to be made. It was acknowledged that more users are now willing to come forward but that they are experiencing a feeling that prescribers don't listen; Prescribers feeling that they "know best" and do not take adequate account of the need of the consumer.

Drinking Reasonably and Moderately with Self Control - DRAMS Scheme

This scheme is presently in use by a number of GPs and whilst it appears to be favoured, it required preparation.

This approach has been adopted by many general practitioners in Scotland. It is based on the evidence that early recognition of hazardous or harmful drinking is possible and intervention at that stage effective. Training courses in the DRAMS Scheme are provided and GPs instructed in the use of a variety of focussed self-help manuals for patients (Gask and Thomson 1990).

REFERENCES

Gask L, Thomson D, DRAMS Scheme: Skills for the General Practitioner. Video and booklets. Scottish Health Education Group 1990.

FORENSIC PSYCHIATRY

D. TONAK

The Council of Europe's statement (early 80s) that "health and criminal justice agencies perceive each other as opponents and engaged in competition over who does what to whom" no longer applies to all parts of the United Kingdom. The change in commissioning management and delivery of health and social care, coupled with a nationally-driven initiative to develop a pro-active approach to mentally disordered offenders (MDOs) has been dealt with in many recent publications, including NHS Community Care (1991), Implementation of the Care Programme Approach (1991), Home Office and Department of Health and Social Services Review of MDOs and similar patients, commonly known as the 'Reed' report, with its 276 recommendations (1992), National Health Service Management Executive priorities and planning (1993) and Health of the Nation (1992).

It was recognised in the final summary of the Reed report that practice all too often falls a long way short of what is desirable. How to meet the shortfalls in both practice and provision was at the heart of that review. In particular it deals with the level and range of provision needed, the mechanisms required to identify and assess the needs of those who should be diverted before entry into the criminal justice system or as soon as possible thereafter and how to ensure effective joint working between statutory and voluntary agencies.

The following **Guiding Principles** should be used as a value base for service developments. Proper attention should be payed to the needs of individuals and to the quality of care they receive. People should be cared for as far as possible, in the community, rather than institutional settings, under conditions of no greater security than is justified by the degree of danger they present to themselves or to others, in such a way as to maximise rehabilitation and their chances of sustaining an independent life, as near as possible, to their own homes and families if they have them.

The planning and development of services must reflect those principles and in order to determine future service patterns there must be regular 'needs assessments', so that agencies can go some way to meeting some of the 276 recommendations in the Reed report.

Assessing need early on is not an easy task because of the NHS and the probation service both being involved with MDOS (see pyramids - diagram 1). This was acknowledged by 'Dr. Reed' who headed the Department of Health, and Social Services/Home Office Review as the most difficult area for assessment - identifying the need for people who pass through the criminal justice system but do not require hospital admission.

The purpose of an assessment of need is to promote and enhance co-ordinated local planning between health, social and criminal justice agencies and this must be identified on a multi-agency basis and become a joint agency responsibility. Health, personal social services and criminal justice agencies have to develop strategic and purchasing plans for services for MDOs.

Needs assessment is the intelligence purchasers require to predict and plan future services. This depends on good quality data - both quantitative and qualitative; while quantitative may be based on assumptions, qualitative may be more meaningful.

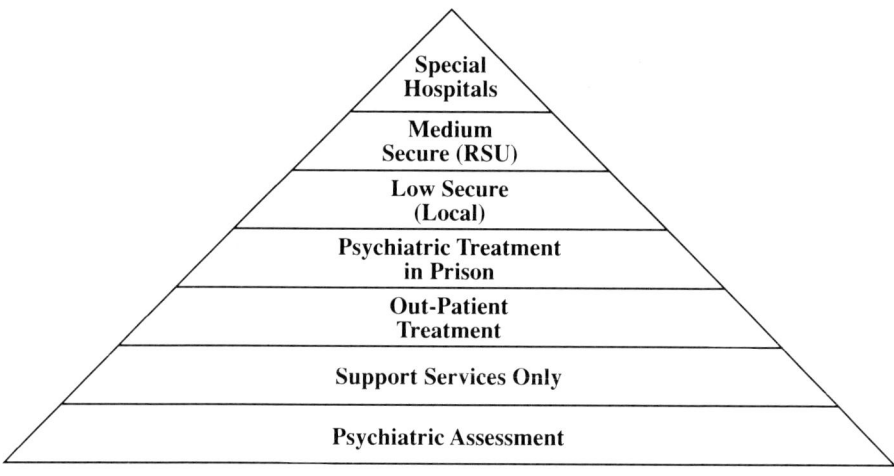

NHS PYRAMID

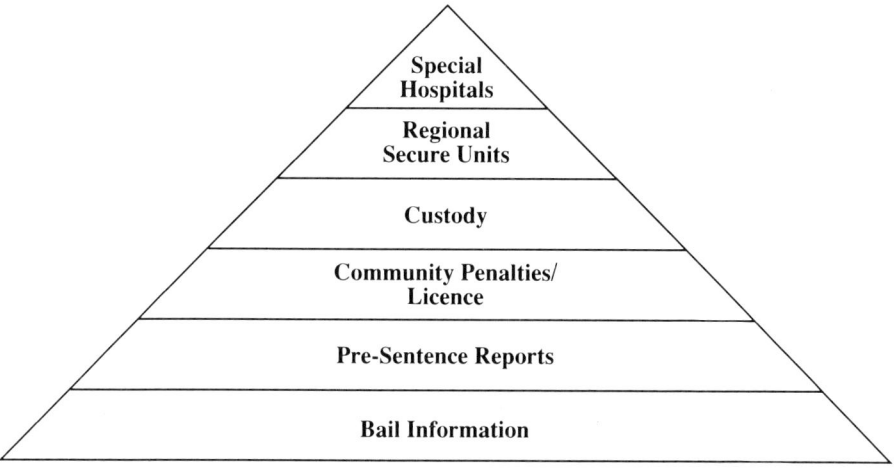

PROBATION PYRAMID

The approach taken in some counties, and a London borough, was to provide a profile of existing day and residential services and usage by mentally disordered people who get into the criminal justice system.

The **quantitative data** about patient activity included the location of MDOs and difficult-to-place patients in the system and the outcome of their placement, whether patients have been admitted from other districts and why and whether MDOs are blocking beds because of lack of appropriate accommodation or lack of social support.

This information, was obtained from: **social services** about the use of community mental health teams of the care programme approach emergency duty teams etc. for MDOS: the **probation** service about the number of MDOs on caseloads the involvement of social/mental health services and the lack of bail accommodation: the **police** about whether they have prompt access to health and social service personnel and whether a policy on a section of the Mental Health Act exists that affects the Police.

Qualitative information is also crucial: this is gained from local multi-agency focus groups, including representatives from the voluntary sector, users and carers. **Focus Groups** provide insights into attitudes, perceptions and opinions. They can identify gaps in services and raise issues causing concern. Information from these groups can be distilled to identify the commonality of need. The quantitative is used to justify some of the points to reinforce the qualitative. Information is analysed and recommendations are made to the local steering committee comprising of health and social service purchasers and providers, senior representatives for the criminal justice agencies. This leads to an agreed joint strategy.

Joint information systems are essential to support joint mental health strategies. Ongoing needs assessments and review based only upon service data is not entirely satisfactory. The use of a local case register will provide valuable information and its establishment is central to the development of joint management and information systems, given the current limitations of national and epidemiological studies.

Diversion and service provision are part of the same equation; there is no point in diverting people from the criminal justice system if services and arrangements are not in place. There are now seventy 'diversion' schemes operational, with as many models as there are schemes. The following are examples of diversion schemes in rural, urban and metropolitan areas.

A Metropolitan Area (Population 700,000) A mental health team, comprising a consultant psychiatrist, community psychiatric nurse, social worker (approved under the Mental Health Act 1983) and a probation officer, is based at the City Court. Health, social and criminal justice (police and probation) agency boundaries are co-terminus in the 8 local sectors around the city. Mentally disordered offenders arrested for an offence are taken to the City Court daily for assessment; the scheme co-ordinator (could be a community psychiatric nurse, social worker or probation officer) in the city is a probation officer who collates information for the team from the person's local doctor, other health and social service personnel or any other agency to whom the person is known, for example, the local multi-cultural organisation.

The decision of the court may be for the case to be dismissed or for the person to be transferred to hospital, voluntarily or compulsorily for either treatment or assessment for the court or put on probation with or without a condition of residence or remanded to a medium secure unit or prison for reports (those cases which are eventually dealt with by Crown Courts which can result in a restriction order to a maximum secure (Special) hospital.

Whatever the decision of the court there is an organisational structure which ensures the mentally disordered offender's key worker is identified and which agency/agencies has/have responsibility for treatment/care/management, etc and is made known to all concerned.

The city prison (for remand and sentenced mentally disordered offenders) has a mental health team and LINK person who liaises with the key worker(s) in the mentally disordered offender's locality. This also applies to medium and maximum secure units.

In each of the 8 sectors the Police has prompt access to a community psychiatric nurse, duty psychiatrist and approved social worker. Those who commit minor crimes are not always prosecuted, when this occurs the local scheme co-ordinator ensures that the mentally disordered offender is "diverted" to a key worker from health and social services". 24 hour crisis intervention units link with local schemes.

Another City   (Population 1.5 million) The City Court houses some 24 courts and may have 500 defendants appearing on any given date.   Community psychiatric nurses examine prosecution papers for those held in custody overnight, before interviewing those who may require a psychiatric assessment - to identify suicide risk, depression, possible psychosis, learning disabilities (mental handicap).   The nurses collate information from the person's GP, social worker, general psychiatrist, etc.   The local consultant psychiatrist and a psychiatrist from the city's medium secure forensic unit and an approved social worker can also attend, if immediate admission under the Mental Health Act is necessary.   All cases are followed through by the liaison Probation Officer, as in the former example.   This city now has a 20 bed hostel for mentally disordered offenders, which facilitates a remand on bail for those of no fixed abode and also provides short term rehabilitation.

A Semi-Rural Area   (Population 350,000) A psychiatric assessment/diversion panel scheme operates through a community mental health team, comprising psychiatric nurse, social worker, a psychiatrist, and a clinical psychologist with access to an occupational therapist, physiotherapist, art/drama therapist, interpreters, and education staff.

A probation officer is co-opted onto this team when information/police/courts/reports on a mentally disordered offender are required.   The probation officer also attends panel meetings to review cases and the team ensure a key worker is appointed from the outset of involvement with a mentally disordered offender (including through and after care from: prison, medium/maximum secure unit.)

A Rural County in Southern England

A community psychiatric nurse, armed with a mobile telephone, is accessible to the police and courts in 3 towns. This CPN has quick access to consultant psychiatrists, approved social workers and probation officers. Links are ensured with the local prison and the county's secure units.

Summary

In order to achieve the aims and objectives of the 1992 Joint Home Office/Department of Health Review of Health and Social Services for Mentally Disordered Offenders, it is vitally important that services in the community are efficient and effective. For this to occur the many agencies involved in providing the comprehensive service required must operate in a co-ordinated way.

While joint approaches to assessment of needs, training and diversion from Custody Schemes have had great value in establishing a solid base for effective inter-agency activity, there is still much to be done in addressing the needs of particular groups such as ethnic minorities, adolescents, women etc.

For those of us who for years have been attempting to effect changes and still consider that changes are slow, should we not bear in mind what F. Scott Fitzgerald wrote in his novel "the Great Gatsby"

"It eluded us then, but no matter - tomorrow we will run faster".

REFERENCES

Department of Health/Home Office (1992) Review of Health and Social Services for Mentally Disordered Offenders and other requiring similar services - Final Summary Report, HMSO CM2088. NHS Management Executive EL (1993) 54 Planning and Priorities Guidance.

HMSO 1992. Health of the Nation - A Strategy for Health in England. ISBN 0-10-119862-0.

FORENSIC PSYCHIATRY

DEREK CHISWICK

Introduction

In the 20 years since publication of the Glancy and Butler reports (Department of Health and Social Security 1974; Home Office and Department of Health and Social Security 1975) there has been a major expansion of forensic psychiatry services in England, and more recently in Wales (Welsh Office 1992). All regional health authorities in England now provide regional facilities for forensic psychiatry; inpatient services are usually based in a regional secure unit (RSU). More recently a joint Department of Health and Home Office (1992) review of services for mentally disordered offenders and others requiring similar services (known as the Reed report) has emphasised the need for a range of services, in both forensic and general psychiatry, to meet the needs of mentally disordered offenders (MDOs). In Scotland there has been no similar comprehensive review.

The remit of the Butler report was confined to England and Wales; it received no proper consideration in Scotland. Barely one year after its publication, two psychopaths escaped from the State Hospital, Carstairs, and murdered three people. A public enquiry followed (Scottish Home and Health Department 1977) and since then government interest in forensic psychiatry in Scotland has centred on facilities at the State Hospital and little else. Indeed, it is not possible to find any comprehensive account of Scottish Office policy in relation to forensic psychiatry services. Any developments have been the result of small local initiatives without special funding (Basson and Woodside 1981).

Psychiatric services in Scotland are changing. Between 1970 and 1990 staffed beds for mental illness fell by 25% while admissions have increased by 38% over the same period. The reduction in beds is likely to continue. It is therefore opportune to consider how services can be provided in Scotland for MDOs and for patients in whom severity and/or chronicity of illness is associated with disturbed behaviour which renders them unmanageable either in the community or in conventional inpatient facilities.

Why is a forensic psychiatry service needed?

Violence is a common feature of psychiatric disorders whether in first-admission cohorts of patients with schizophrenia (Humphreys et al 1992), long stay patients newly discharged into the community (Dayson et al 1992), or residents of hostels for the mentally ill (Marshall and Gath 1992). In any catchment area some patients with psychiatric disorders will present through the criminal justice system. It is therefore necessary to respond to requests for assessment and treatment of people referred by the various elements of the system: police, procurators fiscal, courts and prisons. Each catchment area must also respond to requests from the State Hospital for the transfer of patients who no longer require treatment in conditions of maximum security. All catchment area services must meet these needs but a particular demand falls on psychiatric services for urban conurbations and on services with a prison in their area. In Edinburgh there are approximately 700 forensic referrals to the Royal Edinburgh Hospital (catchment population 0.5 million) each year (see Table 1).

MDOs find themselves at the interface of a variety of agencies and services which have completely different responsibilities and functions. Relationships between these agencies and services are of variable quality. Sometimes they have little understanding of the working practices and problems of other parts of the service (Chiswick et al 1984). However changes in policy or practice in one service (eg increased use of remands in custody for psychiatric reports, or closure of an inpatient facility) will have a "knock-on" effect elsewhere in the system. There are advantages in a dedicated forensic psychiatry service with a single point of entry. In such a service decisions can then be made about the most appropriate service for that particular person. Thus some people will be more appropriately dealt with by a general psychiatry service, others by a forensic service.

Organisation of forensic psychiatry services in Scotland

There is no national strategy for area forensic psychiatry services in Scotland. Some developments have been of a high standard but the overall service is patchy and poorly co-ordinated. With the important exception of the State Hospital, there is no separate funding for forensic psychiatry services in Scotland; services compete with all the other demands in psychiatry for NHS resources. By contrast, protection of budgets has been a feature of regional forensic psychiatry services in England.

There are well established consultant-led forensic services based at the Royal Cornhill Hospital, Aberdeen (Grampian), Hartwood Hospital, Shotts (Lanarkshire), Royal Edinburgh Hospital (Lothian) and the Murray Royal Hospital, Perth (Tayside). These four services all include an intensive psychiatric care unit (IPCU) located within a traditional psychiatric hospital. The service in Glasgow has hitherto been anomalous with a solely outpatient and community service operating from the Douglas Inch Clinic in the city centre. Recently consultants at the Douglas Inch Clinic have established links with IPCUs in the major psychiatric hospitals in Glasgow.

In Scotland IPCUs function as the initial location for patients from courts, prisons and the State Hospital. They should have high levels of staffing. Though they are the nearest Scottish equivalent to an RSU, their physical security is far short of that of an RSU and none of them has been purpose-built. They commonly cater for a combination of forensic and disturbed non-offender patients: the combination is often unsatisfactory. The Mental Welfare Commission for Scotland (1992) reported a wide variation in facilities, admission policies and standards in IPCUs.

Effective follow-up care is the hallmark of a good forensic psychiatry service; it is the most important means of preventing dangerous behaviour by mentally ill patients. There have been developments in some forensic services in community psychiatric nursing, day hospital care and supported accommodation for discharged patients. Such developments depend on "shoe-string" financing and are frequently under threat.

There are currently nine consultant forensic psychiatry posts in Scottish health boards located in Grampian (2), Greater Glasgow (4), Lothian (1) and Tayside (2). All of them are funded partially, and some substantially, by the Scottish Prison Service in return for visiting psychiatrist duties at various prisons in Scotland. In addition there are general psychiatrists with sessional commitments as visiting psychiatrists to other prisons; few of the general psychiatrists have had specific training in forensic psychiatry and some have no involvement in other aspects of forensic work. A forensic psychiatry service is most effective when the visiting psychiatrist to a prison is also responsible for the local IPCU.

The major problems for forensic psychiatry services in Scotland are inadequate hospital and community resources, MDOs inappropriately in the criminal justice system, MDOs in prison, delays in accepting patients transferred from State Hospital and the imbalance between local and State Hospital resources.

Expectations of patients, their relatives, other agencies and psychiatric staff have changed over the years. It is unacceptable for MDOs to remain in prison when they should be in hospital. Patients at the State Hospital who do not require treatment in conditions of special security should not be there. Staff in local hospitals should feel confident that they have safe facilities and proper resources for offender patients and for disturbed patients who prove unmanageable in ordinary admission units. Facilities and treatment in IPCUs (and in other locked wards) should meet the highest professional standards. At present there is wide divergence between the well-resourced facilities of the State Hospital (eg in staffing ratios, accommodation, occupational and social facilities,) and most IPCU's. Yet the risk-taking and labour-intensive stage of patient care is carried out in IPCU's as the patient moves from life behind a fence to life in the community.

Elements of a forensic psychiatry service

An effective service in forensic psychiatry has the range of elements summarised in Figure 2.

It must respond to referrals from a range of agencies; the task is to ensure that mentally ill people receive treatment from psychiatric services. A co-ordinated service with a single point of referral and entry is crucial. This is the most effective way of ensuring early removal of MDOs from the criminal justice system eg by remand to hospital or by direct discussion of cases with the procurators fiscal. Arrangements for dealing with emergency referrals (particularly from the police and courts) are important. A range of inpatient facilities is important so that the type of care is appropriate for the patient's clinical need; not all MDOs need locked wards. Certain attributes in forensic psychiatry staff are necessary. Tolerance for, and sensitivity to the needs of, MDOs and an acceptance of the particular responsibilities in relation to potentially dangerous patients are needed. MDOs are frequently an unpopular group of patients with histories of rejection by general psychiatry services. A capacity to rid oneself of judgmental attitudes in dealing with MDOs must be nurtured in all staff.

Aftercare is of the utmost importance. Most MDOs with a psychiatric illness are already known to psychiatric services and have defaulted or drifted from follow up. Maintaining contact with such patients is one of the greatest challenges facing psychiatry as it moves towards more community-based treatment (Department of Health 1994). In forensic psychiatry the consequences of "mistakes" in this area may be dire. Proper follow up requires staff, resources, sound application of mental health legislation and commitment to agreed policies and practice.

Obstacles to be Overcome

Central government and health boards in Scotland have so far failed to recognise the importance of area forensic psychiatry services. Historically, the usual impetus for change in this work is scandal or disaster (Scottish Home and Health Department 1977; Department of Health and Social Security 1980: Department of Health 1992). Now, as the shift from hospital to community services gains momentum in Scotland, it is vital to ensure that adequate services exist for MDOs and for others suffering from serious mental illness, particularly schizophrenia. Health boards need to educate themselves about the psychiatric needs of MDOs in their catchment areas. There are additional responsibilities on those health boards with penal establishments, particularly remand prisons, in the populations they serve; citizens in prisons have the same entitlement to health care as others.

It is too early to know whether the reforms in the NHS in Scotland (particularly the purchaser-provider split) will ease or aggravate the problems for MDOs. Who is the purchaser of psychiatric care for people in the criminal-justice system? Who is going to ensure effective liaison between local authorities and health care agencies? As bed numbers fall, have planners considered the needs of people with enduring mental illness who require continued highly structured, and perhaps secure, care in hospital? These and other questions must be properly addressed. There is an urgent need for a well informed review of services for MDOs in Scotland, and an indication from central government of its policy.

REFERENCES

Basson J V and Woodside M (1981) Assessment of a secure/intensive care/forensic ward. Acta Psychiatricia Scandinavica 64, 132-141.

Chiswick D, McIsaac M W and McClintock F (1984) Prosecution of the mentally disturbed: dilemmas of identification and discretion. Aberdeen: University Press.

Dayson D, Gooch C and Thornicroft G (1992) The TAPS project. 16. Difficult to place, long term psychiatric patients: risk factors for failure to resettle long stay patients in community facilities. British Medical Journal, 305, 993-995.

Department of Health (1992) Report of the committee of inquiry into complaints about Ashworth Hospital, Volumes I and II. Cm 2028-I-II. London: HMSO.

Department of Health (1994) Draft guidance on the discharge of mentally disordered people and their continuing care in the community. London: Department of Health.

Department of Health and Social Security (1974). Revised report on the working party on security in NHS hospitals. (Glancy Report) London: HMSO.

Department of Health and Social Security (1980). Report of the review of Rampton Hospital (Boynton report). London: HMSO.

Department of Health and Home Office (1992) Review of health and social services for mentally disordered offenders and others requiring similar services. (Reed report) Cm 2088. London: HMSO.

Home Office and Department of Health and Social Security (1975) Report of the committee on mentally abnormal offenders. Cmnd. 6244 (Butler report). London: HMSO.

Humphreys M, Johnstone E, MacMillan J and Taylor P. (1992) Dangerous behaviour preceding first admissions for schizophrenia. British Journal of Psychiatry 161, 501 - 505.

Marshall M and Gath D. (1992) What happens to homeless mentally ill people? Follow up of residents of Oxford hostels for homeless. British Medical Journal, 304, 79-80.

Mental Welfare Commission for Scotland (1992) Annual report 1991. Edinburgh: HMSO.

Scottish Home and Health Department (1977) State Hospital, Carstairs: report of public local inquiry into circumstances surrounding the escape of two patients on 30 November 1976 and into security and other arrangements at the hospital. Edinburgh: HMSO.

Welsh Office (1992) Report of the all-Wales advisory group on forensic psychiatry. Cardiff: Welsh Office.

TABLE 1

Forensic Referrals per year to the Royal Edinburgh Hospital	
* Police	150
* Courts (procurators fiscal and sheriff clerks)	350
* Prison	150
* State Hospital	10
* Social Work Departments	20
* General Practitioners	20

FIGURE 1

Agencies and services involved with mentally disordered offenders

| Courts | | Social Work |

| Police | | Prisons |

Mentally Disordered Offenders

| Community Facilities | | State Hospital |

| General Psychiatry | | Forensic Psychiatry |

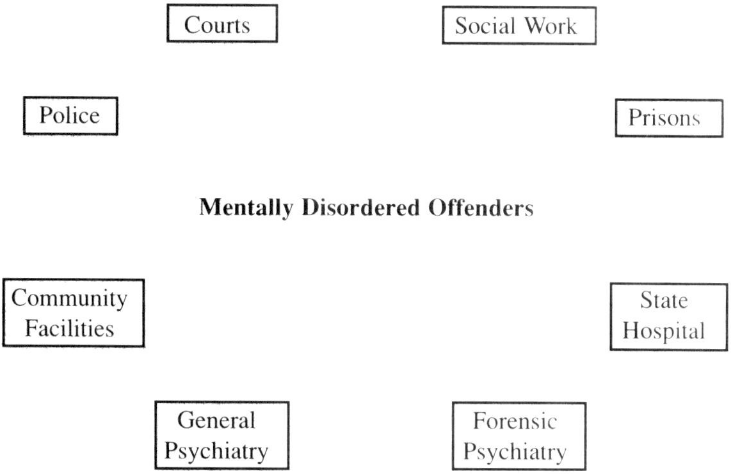

FIGURE 2

Elements of a Forensic Psychiatry Service

* Effective response to requests from police

* Safe, accessible outpatient facility

* Assessment of offenders referred by court

* Effective response to referrals from prison

* Effective response to referrals from State Hospital

* Range of inpatient provision (open ward, IPCU, longer term secure care)

* Access to appropriate community resources (residential and day care)

* Effective arrangements for follow-up of discharged patients

* Multi-professional staffing with secretarial support

INVOLVING SERVICE USER AND CARERS

DR. EDNA CONLON AND JIM REID

The session consisted of a brief introduction from Jim Reid and Edna Conlan in which they indicated that the format of the Session would be nine short presentations entitled "What is Happening Now".

In the introduction it was stated that there had not been enough local user involvement in the preparation of the 1993 Scottish Conference and not enough visibility and involvement of users during the conference. The user voice was not heard at all until the second day and then there were unacceptable time constraints.

There then followed nine Presentations as noted below:-

(1) **North Glasgow Patients Council.** A service user informed the Group about her involvement in the co-ordination of the Maryhill Community Mental Health Council which exists to stimulate self-empowerment and advocacy. Their 1-2 year strategy relates to training, access, respect, trust, value of users, carers and staff. Apparently funding has been agreed from Greater Glasgow Health Board but as yet, has not been received due to administrative delays.

One of the things this group advocates is helping people to assist themselves. It was suggested that people with mental health problems who end up in hospital often have an inherent mistrust of the institution and hierarchy. It was further suggested that there is a need to recognise both sides in setting up new services and that all should work together towards utopia remembering that the users and carers have to use their services.

It was also suggested that medication is a barrier to users' participation and that it would be useful to have empowerment of users by users. The services shouldn't be organised by those with power but should be organised by those who rely on the services.

The speaker also referred to the problem of nurses coming out of hospitals to work in the community and suggested that although you can take the nurse out of the hospital, it may take much longer to take the hospital out of the nurse.

(2) **Bridge Project.** A service user described his work as a full time employee of the

Glasgow Association for Mental Health where he works as a befriender/co-ordinator. Along with the patient administration worker and 15 volunteers linking in with the rehabilitation unit, they organise a range of activities - home visiting, group outings, social activities for those isolated within the community and establish links with health and voluntary organisations.

They also provide support for people in supported accommodation projects and feel that their personal experiences are invaluable in this setting. Most of the long term volunteers from the project are ex-users themselves and they feel that in general, there is a mistrust of professionals. The idea is to build a bridge between the two.

They are also keen to seek out job opportunities and it was suggested that work within Greater Glasgow Health Board could be organised giving them an opportunity to use their experiences of the Health Service to benefit other people.

(3) **Committee of User Representatives (CURE)** A service user described how CURE offers an independent forum for users and carers. The idea is not to impose user groups but to give access to users who can't meet at regular times or intervals. Medical, social and economic models of mental illness are discussed with local authority, Greater Glasgow health board, churches etc, in fact, anyone in a position of power in mental health care. He described how they had written to the Scottish Office regarding the compulsory service order and how the response from the Scottish Office was favourable to their comments. He referred to the 3% quota and employment schemes. He suggested that rather than having high-faluting conversations and partnerships that we should work practically to improve the quality of services.

(4) **MIRAGE Group of Unpaid Carers.** A service user spoke about MIRAGE, (the Mental ill Relatives Aid Group, East End). This is the only group supporting carers in Glasgow and was set up 6_ years ago in conjunction with community psychiatric nurses and social workers. The aim was to monitor hospital discharges 24 hours a day, to avoid homelessness and to set up a 24 hour crisis telephone line. He described how relatives are faced with crisis at home and have no time to try and contact a doctor. Subsequently, they end up telephoning the police who take their relatives into custody. He described further how criminal charges can arise and how mentally ill relatives can be kept in jail. He suggested that the police obviously had no liaison with the hospital and that there was a need for a crisis service.

(5) **Manic Depressive Fellowship (Scotland)** A service user who is a member of the manic depressive fellowship (Scotland) reiterated the need for helplines for carers and users. She then described her work with support groups for users with manic depressive illnesses and their carers.

The manic depressive fellowship (Scotland) has been active for one year providing self help groups. The intention is to provide further services in collaboration with other agencies.

In the year that they have been active, they have doubled the number of support groups from five to ten. Members find the sharing of experiences very valuable in relation to the social network and stigma. She described how because of the nature of the illness, there are long period of remission which allows members to participate. She then informed the group that even although the manic depressive fellowship is a national network, there is no funding.

(6) **United Kingdom Advocacy Network (UKAN)** A service user from UKAN described how user groups are divided up based on what they do individually e.g., some are involved in campaigning work where as others offer practical help or advice.

She expressed the opinion that large organisations need to be localised to allow people to speak for themselves.

The last three speakers were under the title of "Linking and Moving towards Independence".

(7) **Link Clubs and Scottish User Network (SUN)** - users as a valued resource A service user described how Glasgow Link Clubs involve over 100 people. She described how development workers etc have been withdrawn. She then described how they have identified gaps in the service and formed an organisation to try and plug these gaps. Current funding for support workers is though the National Schizophrenia Fellowship.

They are currently looking for jobs for people leaving hospital as well as recreational facilities and the drop-in service.

The Link co-ordinator, assistant and support worker require funding of £84,000.

(8) **Link Clubs and SUN** - Practical-Campaigning A service user who is mainly involved in campaigning as a Link support worker spoke about Link clubs. Concern was expressed that bus passes are not allowed in the community unless people are attending day services etc. He went on to say that this pass is a lifeline for the mentally ill and that in Stirling and Edinburgh people get bus passes. He suggested that although Glasgow is supposed to be miles better; Glasgow is actually miles behind in this respect.

(9) **Link Clubs and SUN** - What is SUN? A service user spoke about SUN, the Scottish User Network which was formed in 1989. Users nationwide felt that voluntary organisations did not appreciate their real needs and instead were concerned with satisfying their own agenda. He stressed that although this conference was being billed as the first Scottish Conference on Mental Health, that the first real Scottish Conference on Mental Health was last year (1992) ie. the Scottish Users Conference. He pointed out that the Scottish Users Conference this year or SUC 2 will be organised in 1993 and invited people to attend provided they could afford £58 entry fee.

The presentations concluded and there followed a Question and Answer Session as detailed below.

Question

(1) How do users overcome the problem of setting up local self-help groups for people who are dependent on the health service and how do they overcome the fear and lack of confidence which prevents people from taking control.

Answer

By having user led groups. Sustaining groups is difficult but this can be overcome by making people aware of the difficulties and by using strong members to prop up others until they gain confidence. Other means are, telephone networking and befriending. As always premises and funding are a problem.

Question

(2) This question related to lack of support for students at Glasgow University and other sites who suffer from mental health problems. The questioner asked if there were any interested parties as often the students have no general practitioners and there was no helpful input from university staff.

Answer

The answer centred around education and promotion of mental health on campuses but the Scottish Office can't say what percentage is spent on promoting positive issues on mental health.

Question

(3) This questioner suggested that the National Schizophrenia Fellowship values user involvement and that legislation now demands it but noted that the training of nurses and social workers doesn't encourage user empowerment.

Answer

The answer to this question was that there should be more training by users as it is their service.

Question

(4) This question was more of a statement criticising the patronising attitude of professionals who did not speak up against the users' views.

Closing Remarks - Edna Conlan

Ms. Conlan summed up by saying that user involvement was not really being encouraged at at the Scottish Conference held in October 1993 and that local users **must** have a voice. She spoke about the courage, humour and pathos of not giving up. She then went on to question whether or not the debate actually happened to allow user involvement and commented that most groups fell apart before because they were based in hospital.

She then went on to say that users' groups thrive on experience sharing and advocacy, getting people to speak up for themselves. She further went on to say that the user involvement at the conference was tokenistic and that people just don't know about the pain and suffering of illness and the strength and pride of local user involvement.

She emphasised the word "local" and suggested again that user groups have to be very locally based. She suggested that were we to look at the world through the eyes of carers for one minute, we would be filled with anger and rage.

In conclusion, she stated that users are not attempting to overturn the services and that we are not involved in a contest. Differences she said are good for debate and that by keeping users out of the planning process, professionals are protecting themselves from the real world.

Lastly, she stated that we all must work together as a family.

SUSTAINING COMMUNITY SERVICES

TOM BURNS

Dingleton Hospital, has provided a community-based mental health service since 1968. This approach to community-based mental health services was used as a useful example to illustrate and raise issues in relation to designing a sustainable community mental health service. The practice in Dingleton [1] has been described before. In many ways it remains in the vanguard of community mental health services despite its age. Recently, the author has conducted a controlled trial of its approach in suburban London [2], [3].

The Dingleton approach is characterised by 3 components; home-based assessment, multi-disciplinary assessment, prompt assessment. In addition, there is close contact with local general practitioners (GPs). The study conducted in London suggests that without loss of clinical efficacy there was a reduction of up to 20% in the need for hospital admission and up to a third of the cost of the service (depending on how it is measured). There was no increase in suicide in the experimental approach.

The study had been conducted because of concern about the role of product champions in previous community mental health service studies. The important difference in the St George's study lay in the use of established professionals with long-term commitment to their services rather than young enthusiasts. Despite the overwhelming evidence in favour of community-based services [4], [5], such approaches have not met with universal acceptance and considerable resistance still exists. Some of the areas of resistance were explored.

Issues

How to propose the service goal. Suggesting the service character in negative terms (eg avoiding admissions) is not successful in the long run. It is more important to stress the positive attributes of the service, ie what characterises its approach rather than what does not characterise it. An example of this would be "offering rapid outpatient access".

Describing the service as "radical" has both advantages and drawbacks. The advantage is the "buzz" created and the interest generated in working for a project. The drawbacks are that in the long term it is difficult to maintain and subject to entropy. Radical approaches may depend on the charisma of the leader who can attract staff who leave when he or she finishes. More importantly, other agencies with whom the team has to work may be put off by this characterisation. Support from surrounding services is clearly needed and any suggestion of grandiosity in the community-based team (especially if linked to exaggerated claims such as a "no bed" approach) can lead to failure of co-operation.

Resistance. The main resistance to sustaining community services can come from professional attitudes. A distinction was drawn between the attitudes of non-doctors (who are on the whole very positive to the approach) and doctors who are much more ambivalent.

Undoubtedly psychiatrists are not universally in favour of community care. Many have worked for a number of years to obtain their current clinical expertise and status and feel this may be affected. They consider that a move to the community or domiciliary work may de-skill them and undermine their status. The de-skilling arises from being unable to control the situation in a way that allows them to use all their expertise. This loss of status is extremely important to psychiatrists. The last 30 years have seen major advances in making psychiatry acceptable to other medical disciplines. Bringing psychiatric services into district general hospitals has been a very public expression of this. There is concern that moving to a more community-based service would break these links. Not only would this affect present psychiatrists but it is speculated that this might reduce recruitment to the speciality which has improved so much in the last 30 years.

Many psychiatrists consider community approaches to be inefficient despite the research evidence. This is probably a reaction to the perceived "low tech" character of the work rather than its overall efficiency. Again, this is a threat to the new-found status of psychiatry within the family of medicine.

Community work, by freeing up old assumptions, can generate a competitive rather than co-operative working environment. Many psychiatrists have experienced themselves as being "under fire" from other professions in the multi-disciplinary team. Whilst from a distance this may seem healthy, it is rarely a pleasant experience for those in the firing line.

Solutions

Despite all these concerns it is unlikely that there will be retrenchment into institutional care. All carefully conducted research to date has found community approaches in mental health care at least as efficient and often more efficient than standard practice. The development of the purchaser/provider split will oblige mental health services to build their services on accepted best practice. A number of possible ways forward were discussed.

Firstly, there was a need for greater professional flexibility. Psychiatrists will need to explore different types of consultant contact to ensure that those members of their profession who are uncomfortable with multi-disciplinary community services can still find professional satisfaction. The Royal College of Psychiatrists must address the needs for training in community approaches in psychiatry much more vigorously. Increased emancipation of patients and their increasing demands on the quality of service will inevitably drive towards improved community provision.

Finally, it was suggested that the recruitment of more women into the higher reaches of the profession would facilitate change. On the whole they appear professionally less competitive and more naturally affiliative.

REFERENCES

1. Jones D. "Community Psychiatry in the Borders" from "Creating Mental Health Services in Scotland" (1987) SAMH Publications, Edinburgh.

2. Burns T, Beadsmoore A, Bhat A, Oliver A, Mathers C. A Controlled Trial of Home-Based Acute Psychiatric Services I: Clinical and Social Outcome. British Journal of Psychiatry (1993), 163, 49-54.

3. Burns T, Raftery J, Beadsmoore A, McGuigan S, Dickson M. A Controlled Trial of Home-Based Acute Psychiatric Services II: Treatment Patterns and Costs. British Journal of Psychiatry (1993), 163, 55-61.

4. Braun P, Kochansky G, Shapiro R, Greenberg S, Gudeman J, Johnson, Shore M. Overview: Deinstitutionalisation of Psychiatric Patients, a Critical Review of Outcome Studies. American Journal of Psychiatry, 138: 6 June 1981, 736-749.

5. Mosher L. Alternatives to Psychiatric Hospitalisation: Why has Research Failed to be Translated into Practice? New England Journal of Medicine, 309 No 25, 1579-1580, 1983.

THE MANAGEMENT OF CHANGE: AN EXAMPLE FROM SOUTH WEST THAMES REGION

GREGOR HENDERSON

"Each locality and those involved as service-users, providers and purchasers must find their own way to resolve complex and inter-related problems. The emergence of comprehensive and appropriate mental health services cannot be imposed as a single blue print from outside or above .... comprehensive services must be developed in each locality".

Tom Butler 1993 in "Changing Mental Health Services - The Politics and Policy".

SUMMARY

Introduction to South West Thames Region

South West Thames Region covers an area from SW London through Surrey to West Sussex on the south coast of England. The population is 3 million and is served by 11 District Health Authorities (DHA's), 8 Local Authorities and 5 Family Health Service Authorities. The region is generally above the national average on socio-economic indicators and is a mixture of urban and rural environments.

Statutory mental health services are provided by 12 NHS units (8 NHS trusts, 4 directly managed units) and 8 Social Services provider units. There are still 7 large old mental institutions with a current patient population of approximately 1200 long stay residents.

There are 25 medium secure beds, 110 close supervision (locked) beds, and an average of one acute bed per 5-7,000 people. There are a number of community resource centres and an average of one community mental health team per 30,000-50,000 population. The overall picture is one of some pockets of excellent comprehensive local services as well as poorly co-ordinated patchy community developments. The innovations achieved to date have been generally reliant on individual provider organisations, both statutory and non-statutory.

There is a general over reliance on in-patient care for people with severe and enduring mental illness and a lack of clarity about the use of community based specialist teams and their relationship with the primary health care sector. There are some areas with a strong voluntary agency presence and there is a developing and increasingly influential service user movement.

The Change Process

In 1991, within the context of the NHS and Community Care reforms, South West Thames, Regional Health Authority (SWTRHA) embarked on a programme of change aimed at developing a comprehensive network of local community focused mental health services across the region. This work formed part of the RHA's 1992/93 corporate contract with each of the District Health Authorities (DHA's) in the region. The corporate contract objective stated that: "By the year 2000, there is to be a network of local community focused mental health services across the region".

Initial guidance was issued, by the RHA, which called for a clear local vision for future mental health services, improved joint working between health and social services, an increased concentration of resources on meeting the needs of people with severe and enduring mental illness in the community and a planned approach to the resettlement of people from long stay hospitals[1].

Developing Local Strategies. The RHA's approach has centred on developing local ownership and commitment to change from purchasers. The main vehicle for achieving this has been the RHA's contract with the Centre for Mental Health Services Development (CMHSD), an independent consultancy organisation. The contract ran from July 1991 to March 1994 and has focused on the development of local mental health strategies in each DHA with follow up implementation work. CMHSD consultants have been working with DHAs and local project management groups in producing local strategies since the autumn of 1991.

The RHA devised in consultation with DHA's, criteria against which these strategies would be assessed[2]. This gave clear guidance as to what was expected from local work. The main areas covered by the criteria were:-

* Evidence of close joint work between health and social services, purchasers and providers, statutory and non-statutory agencies.

* Evidence of shared values and principles underpinning the local strategies.

* Prioritising of resources on people with severe and enduring mental illness.

* Strategies to be based on an assessment of local needs for mental health services and on a review of existing services.

* Evidence of local involvement of service users and carers in the review and forward planning work.

* Identification of outcomes or indicators to be assessed which are amenable to audit or monitoring to evaluate progress in terms of meeting people's needs for treatment and continuing care and support.

* Use of service development models which are based on or backed up by reliable research and evaluate evidence.

* Clear identification of how the strategy is to be financed over the period of implementation for both capital and revenue monies.

Once each local strategy was completed in consultation form it was assessed against the above criteria and comments were fed back in to the local consultation process.

Resettlement from Old Long Stay Hospitals. Another area of crucial importance was that where there was an old long stay mental institution, the local strategy was required to demonstrate how the resettlement of the residents would take place as one part of the strategic change process. Where these institutions exist the ability to transfer the revenue tied up in this type of facility into community focused services whilst at the same time running down the institution is critical to success. Without the release of this money, alternative community based services cannot be created; a period of double running costs to be met. The first step required is to identify the costs of reprovided care and then work with all the purchasers of the institutional care to agree how the additional costs are to be met during the period of transition. This calls for purchasers and providers to work closely and flexibly in agreeing these costs. In South West Thames, the RHA does not top slice the revenue budget of DHA's to create a pool of bridging finance. Instead the onus is on the DHA's within their revenue allocations to determine how best to target their finance. For each institution the purchasers have formed purchasing consortiums to agree the resettlement plans and to negotiate fixed price agreements during the period of resettlement. In this way prices are fixed for an agreed period, including revenue costs.

The work in South West Thames has helped identify a number of steps or a critical path, that can help to achieve resettlement and retraction in a strategic way. These are:

* Agreeing a methodology for individual assessments of current hospital residents between the major agencies, (DHA, provider unit, social services, housing agencies).

* Creating a housing consortium or similar such agency or group of local housing agencies whose task is to re-house people. The principle being applied is that everyone has their own home, their own front door and their own tenancy agreement. It is then the duty of the services to support these principles.

* Identifying the capital and revenue requirements by assessing individual needs and the appropriate housing and support solutions.

* Co-ordinating the use of the capital from a variety of sources for the housing stock between the DHA, Social Services, Housing Associations and the private sector.

* Identifying possible sources of additional revenue ie Social Services, Transitional Monies, Joint Finance, etc.

* Finalising a timetabled plan.

* Setting up a multi-agency project management group with dedicated project workers to manage the process.

The important features of this critical path model are individual assessments of need, specialist housing input and dedicated project management.

Progress to Date

Between July and October 1993, the RHA carried out a "stocktake" of work, by DHA purchasers, to assess the progress being made in strategy work, developing local comprehensive community focused services and to check progress on the planning of resettlements from long stay mental institutions[3]. All DHAS had developed local mental health strategies.

On **future service developments,** the plans, on paper at least, look impressive. The main priorities identified by Purchasers' strategies were more accessible local services, more responsive services to the expressed needs of users and carers, reduced dependence on old institutions for acute, elderly and long stay services, better range of community based accommodation for people with long term mental health problems, higher levels of community based support for people with severe and long term illness, reducing admission rates to in-patient facilities by developing community focused support, seamless service between acute inpatient care, community based secondary care and primary care, and concentrating on people with severe and long term mental illness (community support with acute care and specialist backup).

The **main way of achieving these priorities** which have been identified in local strategies are:

*   Develop local community in-patient facilities (rather than relying on centralised DGU sites) for both adults and elderly people with a mental illness.

*   Improve staffing of community based secondary care multi-agency community mental health teams (with community resource centres).

*   Improve community based secondary care links with primary care teams (to ensure continuity of care).

*   Have one means of entry to the service (assessment team or crisis team).

*   Focus resources on people with severe and long term mental illness.

*   Improve user involvement and the development of local advocacy services and service user groups.

*   Develop partnerships with other organisations (especially voluntary and independent sector organisations) to increase the numbers and range of accommodation options for people.

*   Crisis prevention/intervention services (24 hour services).

*   Respite facilities and "safe" houses.

*   User/lay provided support services.

*   Increase in talking therapies, for example, counselling, psychotherapy (and other

complementary services) - to achieve a reduction in dependence on "medication only" orientated treatments.

* Services and activities that promote growth and provide meaningful opportunities (improved relevance of individualised day activities to work, leisure and personal growth, ie club house models, work co-operatives etc).

On **resettlement** a clearer process for resettlement planning emerged from the responses from purchasers. Agreed resettlement plans for the remaining 7 institutions should be able to demonstrate that they have gone through each of the following 7 main stages:

(i) Individual assessments of need for each resident (involving uses and carers, and social services).

(ii) Developing plans for resettlement and reprovision of services, based on needs identified in the assessments.

(iii) Providing detailed revenue and capital costs to the proposed plans as well as an implementation timetable (preferably in 6 month intervals).

Steps (i) to (iii) to be carried out by provider unit and main purchasers with the involvement of social services (led by lead/host purchaser) to then lead to:

(iv) Demonstration of agreed purchaser support to plans and costs.

(v) Identifying the sources of funding for transitional revenue costs (purchasers, social services funding, etc). "Fixed price agreements (between all purchasers) should be reached at this stage to ensure security of revenue funding during the transitional period. This can be achieved through a purchasing agreement signed by each DHA and monitored by the DHA's.

(vi) Identifying all sources of capital funding (direct allocation, regional capital programme, EFL, private sector capital, housing association capital, loans etc).

(vii) Submitting bids for capital through detailed business cases (submitted by providers).

Throughout the process, project management arrangements should be worked on to ensure that as implementation of the agreed plans continues project management arrangements and staff are in place.

Other key findings on resettlement from the "stocktake" were:

* Purchasers have appeared to have greater control of the resettlement process where they have instigated and led the assessment of individual clients.

* Discontent has been voiced by purchasers where they have not had control of the assessment process and are not therefore fully committed to the outcomes. Working towards standardised assessment between purchasers, providers and social services was called for. A number of purchasers noted difficulty in obtaining information from providers as a source of concern.

* The early involvement of social services departments in resettlement planning was recognised as crucially important by purchasers.

* Purchaser co-ordination is of crucial importance and becomes more difficult as numbers of purchasers relating to each institution increase.

* The "lead purchaser" role, ie, the purchaser with the greatest contract volume, in driving forward negotiation and agreement to retraction costings and proposals is crucial.

* Sound provider management is also essential to maintaining purchaser confidence in plans for resettlement.

* Users and carers are still not - with some notable exceptions - systematically being involved fully in individual assessments and discussion about options for their futures.

Main Areas for Improvement

The "stocktake" exercise also identified the areas that required more attention. These centred round the following 2 main areas:

(i) Improving purchasers and providers abilities to cost the strategies 3-5 years in advance and to identify the required (additional) revenue during the period of transition whilst dealing with other known and unknown calls on budgets.

(ii) Working more closely with GPs and other members of the primary care teams to understand their concerns and to help clarify the relationships and roles of the primary care team and the secondary mental health team(s).

Conclusion

The process reported here in South West Thames has helped to raise the profile of mental health across the region. The local work undertaken over the last 2 years by both those purchasing and providing services has resulted in a number of innovative and comprehensive proposals and developments. The overview presented here highlights the work that has been done to date, the achievements made and the areas that will require continual effort and commitment. The next 3-5 years should see a rapid expansion of local community developments across the region which better meet the needs of local people. The local momentum generated over the last 2 years must be maintained to secure long lasting and beneficial changes for people.

The main factors which seem to be crucial for ensuring the required benefits are strong local ownership of and commitment to change, good local multi-agency working, a well supported, developed and resourced network of local service user groups and self help schemes, shared and well articulated and communicated local values and principles amongst statutory and non-statutory agencies.

REFERENCES

1. SWTRHA. "Mental Health Strategy - Early Thoughts Paper". (October 1992).

2.   SWTRHA Criteria for Assessing Local Mental Health Strategies. (February 1993).

3.   SWTRHA. "Stocktake '93 Report - Assessing Region-wide Development Progress in Mental Health and Learning Disabilities".

References available from:

South West Thames Regional Health Authority,
Directorate of Primary and Community Care,
40 Eastbourne Terrace,
London W2 3QR.

TRAINING PROFESSIONALS FOR WORK IN MULTIDISCIPLINARY, COMMUNITY BASED TEAMS

RONALD J. DIAMOND

What needs to happen for professionals to work effectively in community based services?

Issues are somewhat different in training staff for entirely new services, and for new staff entering existing services where a strong culture has already developed. There are also important differences depending on the previous experience of staff, what staff skills can be used and what previous experience needs to be overcome.

Requirements of a new service:

* clearly articulated mission statement for the treatment programme. This includes a clear specification of who is being treated, and the goals for treatment.

* articulation of the treatment philosophy, including the team's orientation towards paternalism, coercion, and risk taking.

* clear understanding of how the new service fits into the existing treatment system.

* the service needs to be designed to meet the special needs of the target population. This may require staff to be involved in activities outside of traditional practice such as involvement in finding a client housing or teaching survival skills in the community.

Preparation for staff needs to include the development of appropriate attitudes, skills and experience.

Attitudes

a. **Paternalism:** The traditional attitude is that patients are unable to make decisions for themselves and professionals must take care of them. For effective community treatment, staff must realise that patients may need help, but can largely be responsible for their own lives. Treatment must start from the patient's own goals.

b. **Prognosis:** The traditional attitude is that schizophrenia generally has a terrible outcome and that any improvement or change is marginal. It is now clear that all people can grow and change over time, and that the long term outcome is probably better than previously thought.

c. **Outcome measures** - what counts towards improvement. The traditional approach looks at symptoms as the critical measure of improvement. Effectively community based treatment requires a shift of focus to being more concerned with function and quality of life.

d. **Success.** A traditional illness model only counts "cures". A rehabilitation approach counts any improvement in function or self esteem as a success that can be built on for larger successes.

e. **Strengths.** The traditional approach is that the patient's illness overwhelms almost everything else. Effective community treatment requires that the patients strengths are acknowledged, encouraged and taken seriously. "People with schizophrenia are much more human than otherwise".

f. **Risk Taking.** The traditional approaches suggest patient safety is a primary value. Effective community treatment often requires balancing short term risk against long term gains. For example, not all patients feeling suicidal need to be hospitalised.

g. **Treatment Resistant Patients.** The traditional approaches assume that patients must be "motivated" or there is nothing we can do. Staff in new services must be willing to work with patients who may initially not want to "buy" what we want to "sell".

Skills required for effective community treatment.

a. **Comprehensive Assessment**

Learning how to establish rapport with severely ill patients.

Learning how to illicit the patient's own agenda for their life.

Learning how to make a comprehensive psychosocial assessment of a patient, including identifying specific needs that must be met in order for the patient to live a stable life in the community.

b. **Treatment Planning**

Learning how to develop a comprehensive treatment plan that addresses pharmacological, psychological and psychosocial issues.

Learning how to distinguish the goals, strategies, and tactics of both short and long-term plans.

Learning how to include the patient's own goal as a part of the treatment planning process.

c. **Intervention**

Learn required interventions, including specific skill training and the use of environmental supports. This includes both traditional and non-traditional approaches, both individually and within groups.

Learn how to work with families, using a psychoeducational approach.

Learn crisis intervention and resolution: how to stabilise and treat acute disturbed patients in the community.

Learn the indications and side effects of psychotropic medications commonly used.

Learn how to handle counter transference issues in oneself and in other staff.

Learn how to put treatment into the context of the patient's life.

d.   Knowledge of the system

Learn how to work with families and other parts of the patients' natural support system.

Learn how to work with the rest of the mental health system, medical system, and social services system.

Experience required of staff

a.   Working in the community, in the patient's own home and environment.

b.   Working with effective role models.

c.   Being part of a multidisciplinary team

Learn how to share responsibility.

Learn how to use the specific skills of the other team members.

REFERENCES

Factor, R.M., Stein, L.I. and Diamond R.J. "A Model Community Psychiatry Curriculum for Psychiatric Residents". Community Mental Health Journal Vol 24, No. 6, Winter 1988 pp 310-326.

Stein, L.I, Diamond R.J. and Factor R.M. A system approach to the care of persons with schizophrenia. In M.I. Herz, S.J. Keith, and J.P. Docherty (Eds.), Schizophrenia: Vol 5, psychological therapies. Amsterdam: Elsevier Science Publishers. (1990).

MEASURING OUTCOMES

DR. LINDA DE CAESTEKER

The measurement of outcomes is important to different groups within the Health Service. It is important to clinicians and providers as a means of conducting trials and controlled evaluations, to monitor individual patient's care, to evaluate the services they provide and to evaluate the effectiveness of different protocols. Purchasers require outcome measures as a basis for deciding which interventions and services to purchase, to choose between different providers and to allow a more explicit debate about the effective use of resources. Public Health Medicine physicians require valid outcomes to adequately assess the health of the population and the effectiveness of interventions.

Outcome measures will allow service users to choose between different treatment options or different providers, to provide greater feedback to professionals on the effects and impacts of treatment and to provide feedback on satisfaction of services. However there are often low expectations from service users, there may not be alternatives available and there is the "gratitude factor" to consider. Patients may consider the most important factor to be time spent with the doctor and service users may disagree with clinical judgements on quality. There has to be a debate on patient defined outcomes to include aspects of services and interventions which are important to consumers and their carers.

Developing outcome measures is problematic as changes in health status are not always due to antecedent health care. For mental health in particular the impact of health care is but one influence among many. Equally, much of health care is under evaluated and too little use is made of known evaluations. In the field of outcome measures there is the tendency to concentrate on what is measurable and in such a rapidly expanding field it is difficult to keep abreast of developments.

Types of Outcome Indicator

Types of outcome indicator used include mortality, adverse events (complications or re-admissions) clinical assessment, health status score, patient and carer opinions. Examples of work on outcome measures in relation to priority services include the Faculty of Public Health document on Population Health Outcome Indicators for the NHS[1], The Medical Outcomes Study[2], Jenkins[3] work on a system of outcome indicators for mental health and unpublished work from other health authorities and boards. The Faculty of Public Health Medicine report on Population Health Outcome Indicators for the NHS attempted to define outcome indicators which reflect effective health service intervention, based on routinely collected, reliable data. The report highlights that in order to develop outcomes we must first be able to describe the service and its utilisation, describe the underlying level of risk in the population and describe the frequency of the particular outcome of events. The outcome indicators related to mental health services identified are the standardised mortality ratio for death between the ages of 15 to 44 with the underlying cause as suicide and self inflicted injury and with death undetermined whether accidentally or purposely inflicted. The report discusses the difficulty over the legal definition of suicide, the fact that not all deaths with the underlying causes of suicide are preventable and that suicides may be under-reported.

The second outcome indicator suggested for mental health services is the SMR for deaths mentioned as associated with schizophrenic psychosis under the age of 75 years. Other examples of outcome indicators are included below.

Examples of Outcome Indicators

* First admission rates
* Re-admission rates
* Numbers and percentage of crisis admissions
* Prevalence of homelessness in schizophrenic patients
* Employment rates in schizophrenic patients
* Global assessment of functioning scale
* General well-being index
* General health questionnaire
* Reduction in the severity of frequency of problem behaviours
* The achievement of mutually agreed goals for charge
* Improved ability to cope with difficulties
* Improved ability to participate and function
* Clinical effectiveness
* Resource usage
* Referral to other services
* Staff perceptions
* Users' perceptions
* Carers' perceptions
* Levels of carer stress

Discussion ranged over a number of topics. A general perception was expressed that accurate measurement of outcomes was difficult, and sometimes seen as threatening by service providers. The incidence of suicide was mentioned in particular, with the associated problem of knowing whether any occurrence is soley associated with mental illness; it was noted that where the suicide rate was higher in Glasgow than the national average, this might influence its use as a reliable outcome measure - others are being piloted. It was acknowledged from this and other examples raised that some consideration has to be given to the issue of whether a good service might be given with little effect.

Measuring outcomes was suggested as a continuation of clinical research, and this issue was debated. It was noted that while data shows differences between neighbouring health providers, these providers might take various service measures based on their own perceptions of need - outcome measurement is informative, and as an extension to clinical research it can change clinical practice, serving the provider and the purchaser of health care.

The specific issue was raised of using outcome measures in evaluating mental health resource centres, and it was noted that in one instance where a purchaser produced a tender document for a resource centre, the results of submissions were suggested that providers were not only unaware of possible outcome measures, but were also unfamiliar with necessary "Structure" measures, such as catchment area size, the mechanisms for referral, resource allocation and so on. The point was discussed about purchasers and providers "getting together" to develop outcome measurements in common - Dr de Caesteker noted that clinicians' input is essential here, to ensure that these measurements are agreed appropriately.

The issue of using epidemiological studies in determining outcome measures in mental health services was debated, with the possible result of dealing with mental illness as though it can be treated like any organic illness. The comment was made that medical inputs in a mental health service are not necessarily the major factors in producing outputs - social help and care might be more productive. The use of assessment tools in mental health was discussed at some length, as was the necessity to include service users' and service providers' perceptions in developing relevant outcome measurements.

It was generally agreed that the development and use of valid and appropriate outcome measures would require the unequivocal commitment of time and resources ensuring that the provider fulfilled service specifications and people benefitted from it in terms of health and satisfaction with the service.

References

1. McCall AJ, Guilliford MC, Population Health Outcome Indicators for the NHS (A Feasibility Study). Faculty of Public Health Medicine, September 1993.

2. Jenkins R, Towards a System of Outcome Indicators in Mental Health. British Journal of Psychiatry (1990); 157:500-514

3. Wells KB, Stewart A, Hays RD, Burnam MA, Rodgers W et al. The Functioning and Well Being of Depressed Patients. JAMA (1989) 262:914-919.

4. Shanks J, Mental Health Outcomes Project. Department of Public Health, South East London Commissioning Agency 1992. East Anglican Regional Health Authority, Outcomes in Mental Health.

THE CHALLENGE FOR SCOTLAND IN THE IMPLEMENTATION OF COMMUNITY CARE

JOHN HOULT

The planners obviously believe they have come up with a Rolls-Royce model of community care for Glasgow. My first challenge to the plan is that it is already obsolete in a number of areas; our business is constantly altering. In 1965 when I started in psychiatry, people said to me that everything had been changing so much in the past few years that it was difficult to know where we were going at that time, but it would all settle down in a few years and stability would return; there hasn't been any stability in the past thirty years. The field of mental health care has been changing so frequently that change itself is the only stable factor. As the planners were sitting down to draw up the Glasgow plan, developments were happening in so many places around the world that the plan was becoming obsolete before even the pencils were even lifted. The challenge then is this: is the plan flexible enough to be able to be able to adapt to the constant input of new discoveries; of new challenges to the accepted way of delivery services.

Mr. Peter Miller in another chapter mentions how the Richmond Fellowship involves service users in their organisation and how they invites service users to screen the applicants when the Fellowship appoints a staff person. I am wondering why they don't appoint a service user to their staff position? Why not go the next step further? There are places in the United States of America where this is being done, where people who have mental illness are themselves employed as counsellors to help other mentally ill people. Can mental health services in Glasgow rise to this challenge? This example is not meant to be a criticism of the Richmond Fellowship who are probably well ahead of most mental health services in Scotland in having service users participate in their organisation. What is important to convey is that if people think their plan is at the forefront of modern mental health care they are wrong; someone is moving the goal posts back even as I speak.

The next challenge to Scotland is about the very term "community care". Scotland has a great tradition of caring for people, and this is one of the reasons medicine has been such a strong profession in Scotland. It is also one of the reasons why so many Scottish citizens are in mental hospitals, many more than in the State of New South Wales in Australia, which has a similar size of population but far fewer people in mental hospitals. For too long professionals have thought that mentally ill people have few capabilities, and that they must be put away and cared for, because they can't care for themselves: if the person didn't need so much care, and even if the hospitals in which they are cared for are dehumanising, the fact that they got "care" made people feel that something was being done.

One of the problems with professionals giving care to people is that it is they who make the decisions. I went to a boarding school and, like it or not, I had to sleep in a big dormitory, I had to go to meals at the same time as everyone else and I had to eat the same food as everyone else. So I know exactly what the former mental hospital patient meant when he told Alison Peter of Sterling University Social Work Research Centre that after he left the mental hospital, he could "go once a week to Safeways and buy p_t_ and blue cheese". This quote, in her study of people with mental health problems in supported accommodation ("Heaven compared to a Hospital Ward", published by Sterling University), illustrates how important is the freedom to make your own choice about simple things like food; how important it is for the quality of people's lives.

The point in recounting this story is to challenge providers to ask their customers - the people who use the services - what they want; not to assume that professionals know what is best for them, but to actually take the trouble to meet with them and consult with them so that the service offered reflects their needs and their preferences, not what the service providers, think they should have. The Glasgow Strategic Plan for Mental Health, over which purchasers and providers have laboured so long and hard, may have to change its warm caring goals if the service users say that it's not what they want.

There are a number of comments to make about the Glasgow Plan. Firstly, the hospitals; will it be possible to achieve full integration of the hospital component into the comprehensive community services, or will the hospital regard itself as something much more than the rest of the service, will it consider itself as the place where the real treatment happens, whereas the community component is only concerned with follow-up and maintenance? Most of the new community staff in Glasgow will be people transferring out of the hospital the challenge to be faced is to get staff to change their mental set, to get them to regard the hospital as just one of a range of facilities needed for good community care. Can Glasgow get its staff to have a community focus, or will they keep their hospital focus and continue to call the community services "the outreach"? My view is that hospitals really are basically places of asylum, not treatment; they are the place of refuge people with worrying behaviour go to while their treatment takes effect. All the treatment given in psychiatry works whatever the location of the patient; only leucotomy and E.C.T. need the facilities of a hospital, and even ECT can be given as an out-patient. Our tradition has been to have our hospital as the focus of our psychiatric service: can Glasgow change that focus?

I would like to challenge Glasgow about its crisis services, of which the providers have been proudly talking. But will they measure up to what service users who have also spoken at the conference say they want? They have said: "We want services that are available 24 hours a day; we want them to react but we don't want them to over-react and put us in hospital". Will the crisis services in Glasgow be operative for the full 24 hours a day? Will they be able to react promptly? Will they be able to assess a person in his own home, and will they be able to support that person, as much as possible, in his own home until his acute episode subsides? Or will the services be merely a funnel to hospital; the sort of service which "over-reacts and puts us in hospital" because it can do little else. Research in the United States of America[1,2] and in Australia[3,4] shows repeatedly that a crisis service which gives proper support to patients and families gets better outcomes than traditional services, eases the families' burden and is much preferred by patients and their families. Will Glasgow meet the challenge and provide crisis services which are proven to be effective, or will it have a service which falls well short and has little impact?

I want to challenge the plans for day hospitals. Research on day hospitals[5] shows that day hospitals are as effective as in-patient care for about 50% of patients referred for in-patient care. It doesn't really come out significantly better than in-patient care. There are other forms of care which have been demonstrated to be better than in-patient care. This information challenges the view that the day hospital is something which Glasgow should be putting a lot of money into developing. It is rather like buying a Morris Oxford - a car of the 1950s and 60s - in the 1990s, when the new cars are so much better. A comparison, an evaluation, which should be informative is that of a day hospital compared to a 24 hour mobile crisis response service which has the ability to support the patient through the crisis. Another concern about day hospitals is that they often become indistinguishable from day centres. In England I have seen day hospitals which very much resemble the old back wards of mental hospitals, with patients sitting around the perimeter of a large day room, smoking, being bored, doing very little. There is an urgent need to give consideration to the value of day hospitals.

Rehabilitating mentally ill people back into the workforce will be a major challenge for Scotland. Will Glasgow continue the traditional British practice of preparing people for work, but actually getting few people back into work, or will it be possible to make the jump into methods which are now demonstrating that they can get mentally ill people back into competitive employment?

In October 1993, I visited some excellent community mental health services in New Hampshire in the United States where they are helping many people, meeting defined criteria for severe and persistent mental illness, get and keep real jobs. This is no longer an arduous programme of training patients in sheltered workshops or similar facilities. In New Hampshire, the training takes place in vivo, in the work situation. If a mentally ill person declares that he or she wants a job, they are referred to a vocational counsellor who spends a few sessions getting the person's vocational background, finding out his or her work preferences, and then giving practical advice about what to say at the interview, and how to explain long absences from the workforce. After that, the mentally ill person is sent to apply for appropriate jobs, which the vocational counsellor has found by the old fashioned process of pounding the streets; the counsellors build up a large network among the businesses in their district. And even in times of high unemployment, there are businesses which are wanting staff, part-time or full-time; opportunities are always around, they are just harder to find. When the mentally ill person gets a job, he or she receives intensive support in the initial phase from both the key worker and from the vocational counsellor. The person is seen several times daily if necessary, to help them to deal with initial anxieties and with any problems that might arise. Once the person settles in, the help does not need to be so intensive, although it can be increased again if problems occur. An important factor is the instruction to the mentally ill person that if for any reason the job doesn't work out, either because they don't like it, or the employer doesn't like the person in the job, this is in no sense a failure, rather it is merely part of the process of learning which job is best for them There is a lot to be learned from every job trial, which is important to utilise in the next job; the vocational counsellor will then help the person find another job. Utilising this approach, New Hampshire is getting many more of its mentally ill people back to work than anywhere else in the United States. As yet unpublished research[6] undertaken at Dartmouth College Medical School has shown the efficacy of this approach compared to the traditional method which involves training then trying to place mentally ill people in work. The key element is the degree of support offered. There is nothing magic about the method; like all good ideas it's simple, though it involves hard work on the part of the staff. Will you in Scotland take up this exciting new challenge, or will you stick to the safe- but ineffective - methods used traditionally in hospitals but now transplanted to the community.

Moving on to the case management or key worker function, the challenge facing Scotland is how to ensure that staffing levels are maintained. It is important to be able to withstand the financial pressures, the demands to cut costs, that are a feature of all health systems. The key worker system is, I believe, the most important component of care for the mentally ill. The relationship that builds up between the key worker on the one hand and the mentally ill person and his or her social network on the other is the lynch pin of good community care; at the most basic level, it ensures that the person continues to take medication, but at other levels it helps the person gain entry to programmes, work and services that would otherwise not be possible. To do this job effectively, time is important; time to establish the rapport and build up the trust which enables key workers to be effective. And because of this need for time, a staff person cannot be key worker for too many mentally ill individuals. But when money is tight and managers are demanding efficiencies, it is essential to convince them that overloading key workers not only produces poor community care, but by reducing their effectiveness will, before long, also reduce their efficiency. Are the providers in Glasgow ready for this challenge? It won't be long in coming.

There's a challenge to the spirit of innovation in Glasgow and to the ability to change the provider's mind - set. In Denver, Colorado in the United States, I have visited a training programme for service users to become assistant case managers. After three months of formal lectures and a further three months of apprenticeship in the field, the trainees are given certificates for satisfactory completion of the course and are then employed as assistant care managers, working alongside the regular care managers in the Community Mental Health centres. There is an even more innovative scheme in Portland, Oregon, where service users have formed their own organisation which provides care management services for other service users. Does it sound too radical? It is a model which has been around in addiction services for fifty years; Alcoholics Anonymous is not unknown to you. The Oregon[7] programme is being evaluated, and you can read about it in Hospital & Community Psychiatry. Can providers of mental health services in Scotland rise to challenges such as these? Can they make imaginative leaps beyond the traditional types of services? Can they allow mentally ill people to develop their potential, or must people be passive recipients of mental health care?

There are many challenges facing people who are developing Community Mental Health services in Scotland. Challenges to those who work with mentally ill people face to face, challenges to those who manage and administrate and to those who actually suffer from mental illness and use mental health services. The main challenge is whether the brave new era of community care will be little more than a transfer of hospital practices and attitudes to a community setting, or will be a leap ahead of the rest of Britain, introducing programmes and practices which are proven to be more effective and which are preferred by service uses, but which require a major change in everyone's mental attitude. Back in the late 1940's and again in the 1960's[8], Scotland's Dingleton Hospital introduced new treatment approaches which have influenced the whole English speaking world. Can Scotland do it again? Although Glasgow is coming late to the era of community care of the mentally ill, this very lateness gives the opportunity to leap over the rest. Can Scotland once again lead the way?

REFERENCES

1. Braun, P., Kochansky, G., Shapiro, R., Greenberg, S., Gudeman, J.E., Johnson, S. and Shore, M.F. (1981). Overview: deinstitutionalisation of psychiatric patients, a critical review of outcome studies. American Journal of Psychiatry. 136. 736-749.

2. Stein, L.K. and Test, M.A. (1980). Alternatives of Mental Hospital treatment. I. Conceptual model, treatment programme and clinical evaluation. Archives of General Psychiatry. 37. 392-397.

3. Hoult, J. (1986). Community Care of the acutely mentally ill. British Journal of Psychiatry. 149. 137-144.

4. Reynolds, I., Jones, J.E., Berry, D.W. and Hoult, J.E. (1990). A crisis team for the mentally ill: the effect on patients, relatives and admissions. Medical Journal of Australia.

5. Creed, F., Black, D. and Anthony, P. (1989). Day-hospital and community treatment for acute psychiatric illness. A critical appraisal. British Journal of Psychiatry. 154. 300-10.

6. Drake, R.E., Beckel, D., Lounsberry, M. and Fox, T. (1992). Individual placement and support model for vocational rehabilitation of people with severe mental illness. Paper presented at Hospital and Community Psychiatry Conference, Toronto, Canada.

7.   Nikkel, R.E., Smith, G. and Edwards, D. (1992). A consumer-operated case management project. Hospital and Community Psychiatry. 43. 577-579.

8.   Jones, K. (1972). A history of the mental health services. London. Routledge and Keegan Paul.